My Body *Is A* Temple

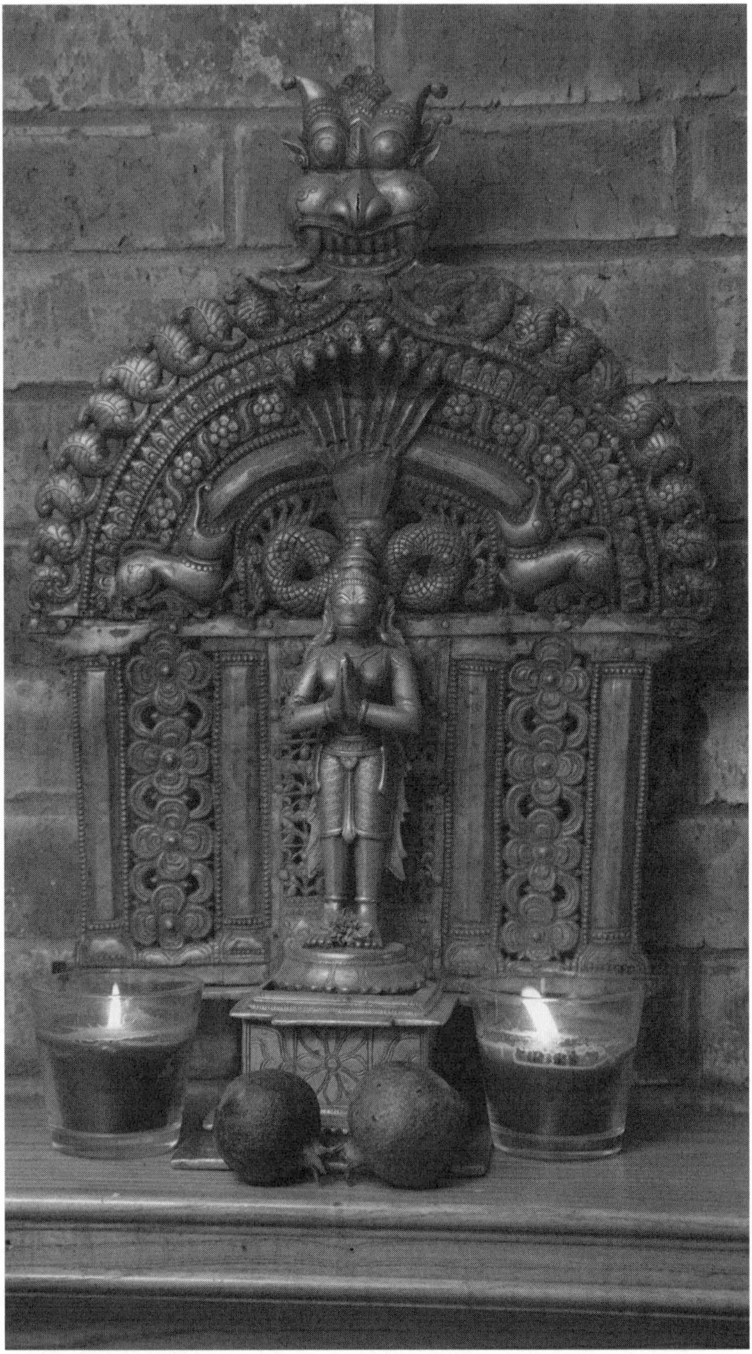

My Body *Is A* Temple

Yoga As a Path to Wholeness

Christina Sell

HOHM PRESS
Prescott, Arizona

Cover Design: Accurance, Bloomington, Illinois

Interior Design and Layout: Accurance, Bloomington, Illinois

Library of Congress Cataloging-in-Publication Data

Sell, Christina, 1969-
My body is a temple : yoga as a path to wholeness / Christina Sell.
p. cm.
Includes bibliographical references and index.
ISBN 978-1-935387-19-0 (trade pbk. : alk. paper)
1. Yoga--Hohm Community. I. Title.
BP605.H58S45 2011
204'.36--dc22
2010046613

HOHM PRESS
P.O. Box 2501
Prescott, AZ 86302
800-381-2700
http://www.hohmpress.com

This book was printed in the U.S.A. on recycled, acid-free paper using soy ink.

To my father, Dr. Michael Frosolono,

for handing me a journal when I was nine
years old, telling me to
“write it exactly like you see it,” and for
encouraging me to write ever since.
Thank you for helping me find my words.

The first glimpse of God has to be in the innermost shrine of your heart. If you have not seen Him there, you can go on talking about Him but you will not ever be able to see Him anywhere. The first encounter has to happen within you.

Once it happens, you will be surprised that you start seeing God everywhere. Once you have seen Him within your heart, how can you miss Him—because everywhere the heart is throbbing with Him. The tree is full of Him and the rock also, and the river and the ocean, and the animals and the birds, everywhere. Once you have felt His pulse, once you have felt Him circulating in your own blood, once you have had an experience in your own marrow, then everywhere, wherever you look you will find Him. But it cannot happen otherwise. If you are empty of His experience, you can go to the farthest corner of the world; your traveling will be in vain. If your own house does not become His temple, then no temple can be His abode. If your own house has become His temple, then all houses are His abode.

—Osho

Acknowledgements

Like any worthwhile endeavor, writing a book is a community effort.
I extend my heartfelt gratitude to:

Yogi Ramsuratkumar for building His temple so that I might learn to build my own.
Lee Lozowick for teaching me what it means to be Loved.
John Friend for your unbounded personal and professional support. And for Anusara Yoga. Seriously. Wow.
My sangha mates for showing me every day what it means to stay in place.
The Anusara Yoga kula for the laughter, the tears and the nectar of Good Company.
My husband Kelly, for believing in me and for believing in us. And for showing me that both are worth fighting for.
My teaching partners and brothers on the Path, Darren Rhodes and Noah Maze. Your friendship is a blessing. I am who I am today because of both of you.
Elena Brower for the ongoing conversation, and for teaching the world that beauty is a state of mind and heart.
Christy Nones for your skillful and careful editing of the initial manuscript. Your passion, precision and clarity was a boon.

My editor and mentor Regina Sara Ryan for patiently guiding me through the process of bringing this project to completion and for your unrelenting enthusiasm for the subject matter.
Gioconda Parker for becoming my friend when I really needed one. I think you may have saved my life.
The Lemons on 6th and Lamar for making my life a whole lot more fun this year.
My yoga students everywhere who have taught me most of what I know about teaching yoga.

Thank you for sharing the journey with me.

Contents

Foreword

I wholeheartedly recommend Christina Sell's *My Body Is A Temple*. Not because I happen to be her Teacher but because her common sense wisdom, immediately pragmatic instructions (or at least suggestions) and heartfullness in her care and compassion for the well-being of others, any and all others, oozes through the words like pure maple syrup. We live in a troubled world and to blame the world's ills on all those "out there," neglecting our own contribution, even if our own contribution is avoidance of the issues, detachment through self-absorption, or simply a critical overview that obstructs our involvement, certainly isn't of much value. We, the world, is an interconnected whole, a symbiotic field of mutual influence, inter-dependence and oneness. We cannot help but be a part of this field, like it or not, active or passive, even knowing so or not. When any one of us comes to a "higher" understanding of Reality, as-it-is, here and now, all of us benefit. So this book is not about some exclusive spiritual path or practice. It is about each and every one of us. You, me and everyone. The principles that Christina has devoted her life to are universal, meaning that they not only apply to all of us but can, and will, given even a small chance, benefit all of us.

The body as temple, the heart (or another word in this context could be *soul*) as shrine, could have come from, in slightly different language but no difference in meaning,

Buddhism. Judaism, Christianity or any other number of sources. As I mentioned just before, these principles are quite universal. So please do not get hung up on the language but read and feel deeply into the essence, the spirit of Ms. Sell's wonderful and delicious offering here in these following pages. And remember, but only if you wish to, that without active practice, the integration, digestion and demonstration in our lives, of the information presented here, you might at well consider this book just another diversion, a pleasurable romp through the spring flowers, but of no actual benefit. So as she titles one of the sections: "practice, practice, practice." And I might add, most likely unnecessarily echoing the author's words, that it doesn't pay to be impatient. Like a seed planted in rich earth, and do consider yourselves rich earth with profound possibility, time is not just required but is a natural aspect of the coming to fulfillment of that seed, time for it to germinate, poke its delicate head above ground, grow to maturity, and with the proper nutrition, water, sunlight, the chemicals of the earth, and care or protection from damage or predators, essentially produce its fruit, flower or vegetable. So give your body and heart (soul) a running start, a chance to allow your diligent practice to blossom and shine. Thank you!

—lee lozowick
Prescott, Arizona
May 3, 2010

PREFACE

This book is the result of the influence of my two primary teachers—Lee Lozowick, my guru and John Friend, the founder of Anusara Yoga. I met these two extraordinary men within six months of each other and have had the good fortune to enjoy an ongoing and ever-deepening relationship with them both. Over the years their relationship with one another has evolved into one of mutual respect and admiration, which serves as a source of delight and inspiration to me and those who know them. Without the help of these two teachers I would have little to say on any topic related to yoga and spiritual practice. Additionally, this book references Carlos Pomeda and Professor Douglas Renfrew Brooks, with whom I have periodically studied yoga philosophy

In *Yoga from the Inside Out* (Hohm Press, 2003) I presented many of Lee Lozowick's primary teachings alongside the teachings of Anusara Yoga in a way that was consistent with my personal practice and direct experience. While Lee Lozowick teaches in what he calls the "Western Baul tradition," and John Friend's Anusara Yoga philosophy is informed by the elegant philosophies of Northern India (Kashmir Shaivism, primarily) as well as Southern Indian schools such as the Shri Vidya tradition, their schools are, in my opinion and experience, more complementary than different.

At the heart of each tradition is the recognition that there is one singular presence behind all manifestation. Both traditions invite the yoga practitioner into a direct and personal relationship with this singular presence through the radical affirmation of life *as it is*, within a community of like-minded practitioners, and under the guidance of a skillful teacher. Both traditions teach in practical ways how we might rely on the Divine and its blessings in the midst of the challenges of our ordinary lives.

This book is not intended to be a treatise on either the Western Baul or the Anusara Yoga tradition, nor is it intended to be a synthesis of them. My intention is to outline basic principles of spiritual practice as they relate to a variety of disciplines, and to show how people of all faiths and practitioners of all methods of yoga might see and experience those endeavors from the highest possible perspective.

Any mistakes I have made in this presentation are due to my own ignorance and inexperience. Truly, anything useful belongs to the wise and compassionate teachers who have so generously guided me. May the influences of the different lineages that inform this offering guide each one of us along this ageless path of learning, transformation and awakening called yoga.

—Christina Sell
August 2010

Introduction

Time was when I despised the body;
But then I saw the God within.
The body, I realized is the Lord's temple;
And so I began preserving it with care Infinite.

—Bhogar (circa 1600)

The body as a temple is a common metaphor in many spiritual schools and traditions. As a person who has battled body image and food addiction issues for much of my life, I have always been struck by this metaphor because of the difficulty I have had accepting my own body. For many years, the vision of my body as a temple, though inspiring, was much too grand for me to actually relate to and put to practice. Before embodying such a context, I had to first end a war I had been waging against myself and my body, and make peace. *Yoga from the Inside Out*—which I wrote in 2002—describes a process of making peace with my body that occurred through the application of spiritual precepts under Lee Lozowick's direction and through the principles and practices of Anusara Yoga. As the years have passed, and I have become more established in a relationship of peace with myself and my body, I realized there was a step to take beyond "making peace." This next step took me into the domain of discipleship and spiritual life, where I began to see that a life of spiritual practice is a type of sanctuary in and of itself. Practicing according to the deepest truths of the heart is its own refuge. This lifestyle helps the practitioner cultivate a physical body that is stable, bright, and thus able to withstand the rigors of service, devotion and transformation.

Although I have always loved the idea that the body is a temple, this idea came to life for me on my first trip to India in 2004, in the company of my spiritual teacher Lee Lozowick and a group of his students. This trip was a pilgrimage in many ways, because it included a visit to the ashram of Lee's guru, Yogi Ramsuratkumar, an Indian saint who spent most of his life in southern India in Tamil Nadu. This trip was an opportunity for my teacher to visit the sacred ashram of his master, and for those of us who were Lee's students to glimpse the *parampara*, the lineage, of which we are a part.

After a long, sleepless, intercontinental flight, and a harrowing bus ride that I was soon to learn was quite typical of bus rides in India, our bedraggled traveling group arrived in Tiruvannamalai in the shadow of the sacred mountain Arunachala, and proceeded immediately to the Yogi Ramsuratkumar Ashram, where we spent four days participating in their programs. With this as our base we explored the town and neighboring ashrams. Being in India was exhilarating, deeply healing and inspirational. Many of my preconceived ideas about "the Path" were overturned in the process, and my ideas about what a yogi *is* were redefined here. Despite the fact that Yogi Ramsuratkumar had left his body in 2001, the time at his ashram was the highlight of my five weeks in India. Here we had the opportunity to meet with Ma Devaki, who had been Yogi Ramsuratkumar's personal attendant since 1993.

In some of these meetings, Ma Devaki told us stories of her life with Yogi Ramsuratkumar, including the many miracles she experienced in his company. She told us about his adamant claim that his ashram was sacred ground where, as he said, "anyone who came would be blessed." She told us about how his temple was built, and how he intended it to be the means by which he would continue to impart his blessings after his physical body had passed. In those conversations with our group she repeatedly asked us, "Do you feel Him him here?" I remember always answering affirmatively. "Yes," I told her, I felt him. And although I was deliriously happy during my stay at Yogi Ramsuratkumar Ashram, quite frankly, I answered "yes" mostly to be polite.

Several days after leaving Tiruvannamalai, our group visited another temple in Tamil Nadu. I remember that the architecture and the iconography were stunning. I also remember that there was a distinctly different quality to my inner state at this temple. I found that I felt less happy there than I had at Yogi Ramsuratkumar Ashram. "Was that supremely happy feeling that I had felt actually Yogi Ramsuratkumar's blessing?" I began to wonder. "Had his temple actually been able to transmit to me the blessing of this hidden saint, just as he said it would? And could it be that those blessings would actually come to me from within, in an experience of inner joy, deep happiness and exquisite satisfaction with the life I had chosen?"

I pondered these questions throughout the remainder of the trip, and also noticed that certain practices would re-create the same state of being—or a close approximation—to what I had experienced sitting in Yogi Ramsuratkumar's temple. Chanting, *asana*, *pranayama*, meditation and even visualization could recreate within me a happiness similar to what I felt there. This book is a result of my ongoing wondering about whether or not asana practice was a means to build a place of worship within myself. "Do the forms of practice embody the necessary building blocks to construct a life that is a sanctuary and a body that is a temple?" I asked myself. Could a life of practice help me to abide more constantly at the shrine of my own heart?

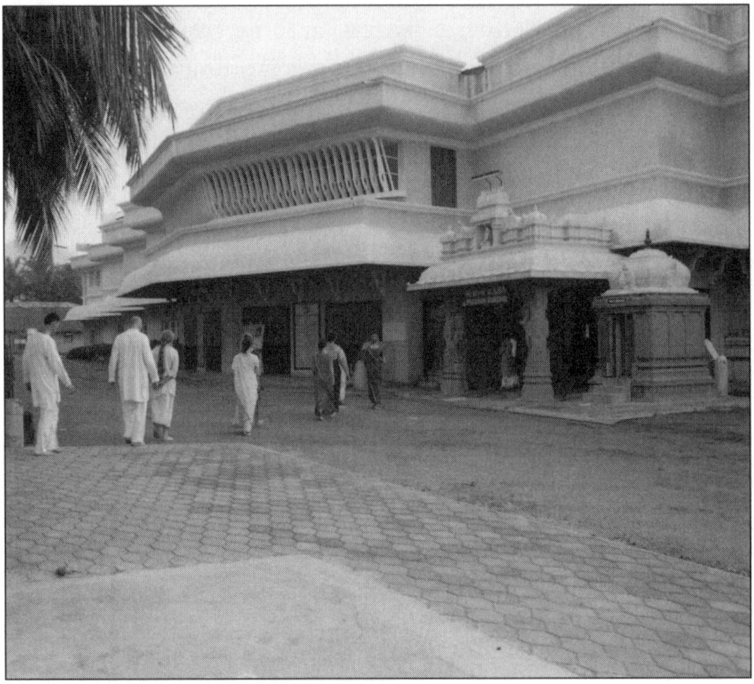

Western devotees approach the Temple of Yogi Ramsuratkumar, Tiruvannamalai, South India, Winter 2005.

As I have become more passionate about these ideas of building a temple of the body, I have continued incorporating them into my practice and into the classes and workshops I teach. I have found this metaphor rich, engaging and relevant to my own practice. Students from many traditions also seem to relate to this idea and make use of the metaphor. I really cannot say that I have fully embodied this teaching, as obviously I am still very much a work in process. Success in yoga is not measured easily, nor is it measured in the short term. However, I can testify that when I practice with high ideals such as these, I am called into their higher sphere for my points of reference, rather than remaining in the sphere of my habitual, ordinary mind. Living in a sphere other than my habitual mind makes all the difference in the world to me. Rather than just performing the asanas physically, I practice the asanas as a means to embody these high ideals. In doing so, my asanas become prayers, affirmations and gestures of remembrance.

This conscious fusion of the physical with the metaphysical, and the commitment to explicating that relationship, is one of the hallmarks of practicing yoga as a spiritual art. By "physicalizing virtue," a yoga practitioner uses asana as a decidedly spiritual endeavor. This approach has been profoundly transformational for me, literally changing how I see myself, how I view the world around me, and determining what I think about. Practicing yoga as a spiritual art has delivered me to a different state of consciousness, one that would have been impossible to achieve through the mere repetition of physical gestures. The practice has aligned my attitude as well as my body.

Building a temple of the body is a metaphor meant to inspire our efforts in yoga toward a higher possibility than simply "stretching and strengthening" or even "being happier" or more "centered." Building a temple of the body is hopefully an instruction manual for dedicating oneself to a life of the spirit in and through the vehicle of the body. Interestingly, there are ongoing debates in the world of yoga philosophy about whether the body is a "vehicle of consciousness" or whether it is an "expression of consciousness." But these distinctions are outside the scope of this book. However, on a more personal note, one evening I tentatively asked my spiritual teacher, Lee: "Is the body a vehicle of the Divine or is it an expression of the Divine?" He rolled his eyes, sighed heavily and said, "It depends on the day."

If we look at Yogi Ramsuratkumar's temple as an authoritative example, then the body is both. The body, as our temple, is both the house of the spirit and the spirit made manifest. Why spend a lot of time dividing it all up? In fact, as sincere seekers we can find the value in both vantage points, seeing each perspective as an important facet of the diamond of an inclusive view.

Certainly for yoga scholars and students of comparative religion, these distinctions are important. I am neither. What I am is a sincere student of a great art called yoga, which rewards my progress on the path with increasingly difficult challenges. I am a fumbling yet dedicated student of a force of grace called Yogi Ramsuratkumar, as it is embedded in the vehicle called Lee Lozowick, my spiritual teacher. As his student, I am constantly challenged to say yes to the seemingly impossible, and then to rely on that very same force of grace to show me how to fuel my efforts optimally. Truth be told, I am basically a spoiled, neurotic, American woman who is drawn to Eastern contemplative practices like meditation, prayer, asana and mantra as much as I am to shopping malls, fine restaurants and nice clothes. I am not a renunciate, a scholar or a yogic expert. This book is not concerned with ironing out the nitty-gritty details of yoga philosophy. Nor is this book intended to be an exhaustive treatise on hatha yoga, asana practice, yoga philosophy or my teacher's ministry.

Instead, this book is an invitation to each of us to engage a great temple-building project of our own. We can create a life of practice that builds a great temple of the body that will be both a vehicle for, as well as the literal embodiment of, grace. This book is meant to encourage and inspire each of us to enter fully into our lives here, now, however we find them, with the assumption that our lives contain within them a Divine blueprint for success, and all the bricks, mortar, raw materials and energy necessary to build a great temple. We *can* cultivate ourselves through yogic practices to become a temple that can provide refuge and sanctuary so that we might serve something greater than our own personal whims.

The Structure

My Body Is a Temple, Yoga As A Path to Wholeness is organized around six basic principles and utilizes the metaphor of building a temple of the body as a way to bring the principles of practice alive in a meaningful way. The six principles are 1.) Building Plans: Put the Highest First, 2.) Foundations: Establishing a Solid Foundation, 3.) Scaffolding: Erecting and Maintaining Strong Walls of Support, 4.) Entering the Sanctuary: Expanding the Inner Life, 5.) Worship: Life at the Shrine of the Heart, and 6.) Outreach Ministry: Service and Celebration.

The philosophies that inform my yoga practice suggest that the physical world is a microcosm of the spiritual. The physical world, the world of matter, is seen as condensed spiritual energy that functions according to the same principles as the world of the spirit. The theory follows that by understanding one end of the spectrum, one may gain entry into or understanding about the other. Given these philosophies of totality, many metaphors could be put to use in a book like this. The temple of the body is certainly not the only useful metaphor, but one for which I have an affinity due to my love for Yogi Ramsuratkumar and his temple, and because of my own struggle to love, honor and respect my physical structure as a temple.

At the end of each chapter I have included questions for contemplation. After I wrote *Yoga from the Inside Out*, many people asked me, "But how do I actually *do it*? How do I actually take this starting point of a 'war with the body' and actually 'make peace'? How do I start with self-hatred and transform it into self-love?" I received as many letters thanking me for sharing my story as I did requests for more tangible, practical advice. Evidently, I had failed to make clear that much of the transformation happens internally, in the midst of ordinary circumstances, and that there is no easy way to bring these principles to life. No teacher, no class, no book, not even any particular yoga method can do the work for us. However, writing and discussion are great tools that can help these ideas come to life inside each of us. Only by taking an idea and chewing on it awhile can we internalize and be guided by it. This book is intended to provide food for thought that will most definitely require some chewing. It is in no way intended to offer a simple solution or a quick fix.

Ways of Knowing

In the first chapter of the Yoga Sutras of Patanjali, Patanjali discusses something called *pramana* or "correct knowledge." He says we can know correct knowledge in one of three ways: 1. *pratyaksa*—direct perception, 2. *anumana*—inference and 3. *agama*—scriptural reference or the testimony of an expert of scripture.[(1)] When inquiring into the nature of the Divine and the means by which we might align ourselves with it in order to build a temple of the body we will rely on these three primary ways of knowing that Patanjali outlined.

1. We will rely on our own direct perception, *pratyaksa*, including those situations where our "hair stands on end." These are moments of recognition, and we will rely on them as markers of truth. We will use those feelings of deep rightness and inner alignment that tell us we are close to the truth. We will learn to rely, over time, on our intuition and on our past experiences.

Yoga philosophy comes from a long history of debate and argument. Personally, however, I have little interest in debating matters of faith. To the extent that a philosophy serves to deepen one's faith in that which affirms life and beauty, I believe that philosophy is a wonderful thing. But if any philosophy presented in this book interferes with your chosen faith, with your own direct perception of truth, then feel free to regard the ideas presented as simply that—as ideas.

2. We will utilize inference, *anumana*. This is the idea that "where there is smoke there is fire." For instance, in building a temple of the body, we might begin to see that longstanding injuries heal when we practice in optimal physical alignment. We would rightly infer that we are in alignment because when we are in alignment our pain diminishes. But we also have to be careful about any inferences we make. As we mature in this process we will make more appropriate distinctions. For example, the mature practitioner appreciates that discomfort is not necessarily a bad thing. Sometimes strong sensation is necessary for transformation. Sometimes, the most optimal way to do a pose creates intense sensations that the unseasoned practitioner will label as "painful." To infer that this type of pain, which is actually just strong sensation, was signaling something incorrect would not be accurate. We can learn to distinguish pain from sensation and, over time, learn to infer and perceive which sensation is optimal alignment and which is deleterious.

In the process of "right alignment," sometimes we will uncover painful emotions, or go through periods of sadness and inner turmoil. It would not always be accurate to infer that, because we had a less-than-enjoyable feeling state, we were out of alignment with the Divine. Once again, it is imperative that we learn certain guiding principles and how to make appropriate distinctions for them to be truly useful to us.

3. We will rely on testimony, *agama*. We will review philosophy from different traditions and rely on the testimony of people who are authorities on yoga and spiritual traditions. This means of knowing can be problematic in our culture, where abuses of power are commonplace and where authority is either blindly followed or recklessly ignored. When relying on testimony and in determining what is authoritative, each one of us needs to be both open-minded and scrutinizing. This essential balance could be the subject of its own book, and we will certainly talk more about it when we get to Chapter 12, in which we consider gurus and teachers.

How to Use This Book

Use a journal as you read this book. If you do not already own a journal, please buy one for yourself. Get a pen that you love to write with. Do whatever you need to do to assist yourself in actually doing the suggested writing exercises. Decide to explore the questions and concepts I have written about as you read. There are numerous ways to do this. I suggest that you look over the questions at the end of each chapter and consider them. Take your time. Choose one and write about it as often as possible over the course of a week. The following week, choose another one that most interests you. Or invite a friend to read the book with you and do the exercises as well. Then the two of you could get together to discuss your discoveries. Or you could start a group in which you consider one question or concept each week: write about, discuss it, and thus begin the processes of bringing these ideas to life.

Eat the Meal

While philosophy can be inspiring and certainly help us to align our efforts with certain perennial truths, philosophy without practice is relatively meaningless. One of my philosophy teachers, Carlos Pomeda, is a rare combination of spiritual practitioner and scholar. He has devoted thirty-four years to spiritual study and practice, living many of those years in the Siddha Yoga ashrams. Additionally, he holds degrees in religious studies and Sanskrit. He told me once that "knowing the philosophy without doing the practices is like being able to read a recipe in a gourmet cookbook but never getting to eat the meal."(2)

This book is about getting to eat the meal. If any of the philosophy is at all interesting, I implore you to put it to practice. If the idea that each one of us can build an interior temple that not only sanctifies the body but establishes a "body of prayer and devotion" is appealing, then please begin to practice accordingly. Make it your number one priority to bring these ideals to life. I cannot imagine a better way to spend one's life than pursuing such a vision. My hope is that the information here is basic enough for the new practitioner to find useful, and deep enough that the experienced yogi will find clarity and fuel for ongoing practice.

May Yogi Ramsuratkumar's blessings inspire these writings and these considerations the way they inspired his temple. May his blessings help each one of us to enter more fully into the domain of inspired practice and to live more fully in joyful service to the flow of the Divine. May each one of us build a temple of the body. May each one of us learn to worship at the shrine of our heart. May each one of us have great company along the way.

Questions to Consider and Write About

1. Does your life in action show that you trust your own direct experience or the testimony of spiritual authorities more?
2. How do you recognize your direct experience of truth?
3. What makes testimony reliable?
4. What do you mean by “an authoritative spiritual source”?
5. Who or what is an authoritative spiritual source for you?

PART I

BUILDING PLANS: PUT THE HIGHEST FIRST

I have often heard my spiritual teacher remark that "context is everything" when it comes to spiritual life. An optimal context for yoga practice involves joining our intention, attention and efforts in the aim of our heart and learning to see and live from that perspective. This first part outlines many of the concepts that govern the spiritual context for building a temple of the body.

one

Intention

The shortest distance between two points is intention.
—Randolph Stone, Polarity Therapy

Shoot for the moon. Even if you miss you will land among the stars.
—Les Brown

The Sanskrit word *samkalpa* means "volition" or "intention." Yogi Ramsuratkumar started his temple-building project with an inspiration, with an intention or samkalpa for his temple. He wanted his temple to serve as a place of pilgrimage and as a means of transmitting his blessings after he was no longer in his physical body. Repeatedly, and over a long period of time, he clearly stated his intention that, "Anyone who comes to my ashram and anyone who comes to this temple will be blessed."

So too, we begin our efforts of building a temple of the body with an inspiration and intention that reflects our deepest reasons for our endeavor. The use of samkalpa allows us to consciously connect our physical actions to our highest ideals. By clarifying our samkalpa, our intention serves to channel the will we bring to our practice, and helps us connect our personal desires to a larger process of awakening.

Why We Practice

Many people come to yoga practice with an ordinary inspiration such as "I want to be more flexible" or "I need to calm down" or even "I want to get fit." Others come for the more "spiritual" promises like inner peace, greater compassion and expanding one's consciousness. And while the exterior reasons vary a bit from person to person, most of the reasons boil down to, "I have a longing to know myself more fully. I want to experience a greater freedom and live from that knowledge. I think yoga can help me somehow."

Sometimes, without even realizing it, we fall into the trap of thinking our own individual reasons for practice are superior to others. Instead of looking for the unity that underlies our efforts, we can get caught in the apparent diversity of motives. A favorite pastime among some yoga practitioners of various methods is to criticize other people's motives for practicing yoga. The physically-demanding traditions scorn the "fluffy" reasons for practice, saying that "You cannot have inner peace if your body is weak and toxic. Forget about all that woo-woo stuff and just handle the body." The more mystical traditions say, with equal scorn, "Those people with their physical yoga are just doing gymnastics. It isn't real yoga."

These conversations and discriminations remind me of my zealous environmentalist friends from college who were upset that people were only recycling because it was suddenly a "cool" thing to do, not because they really cared about the Earth. I kept thinking, "Who cares why people are recycling? They are recycling. Isn't that what you wanted anyway?" In the same light, I do not concern myself so much with the overt reasons *why* people are practicing yoga because I see the different motivations as facets of the same diamond: as various manifestations of the longing to align with our intrinsic samkalpa, to experience a greater freedom and self-knowledge and to act from that understanding. Wanting to do something good for ourselves—like yoga—simply aligns us with that fundamental part of us that *is* good and knows that we deserve "the goodness" of health, clarity, integrity and happiness. And if, as our yogic philosophy suggests, the body is a microcosm of greater spiritual forces, then wanting health of the body is not divorced from spiritual intention. When we are building a temple of the body we want the structure to be sound, laid out according to a solid plan, and built with the best construction materials and technology available. Physical fitness, it seems, is no longer such a lowly intention. Seen from this perspective, freedom for the body is freedom for the heart. Whatever gets (and keeps!) someone on the path of yoga is great because every motive points us back to our heart's intention, to our samkalpa, to experience a higher degree of freedom and self-knowledge.

Down to Earth

Even the loftiest of intentions must be brought down to earth, brought to life in the messy and humbling domain of human experience. One of my counselors in college used to tell me all the time, "You know, Christina, you just can't get through life without getting some of it on you!" Even the most transcendent of aspirations must be made quite real in this endeavor of temple building. Otherwise, it makes no difference.

Building a temple of the body is as much an intention *for* practice as it is an outcome *of* our practice. This intention places our attention and efforts in a stream of extremely high ideals. Many people are afraid to aim high and to set bold intentions. Many do not, deep down, believe it is possible or believe they are capable or worthy of realizing such aims. Nevertheless, the very idea of samkalpa is that we aim high. The spirit of samkalpa in building the temple of the body is that we establish the intention to align our efforts with our highest possibility and then get to work on the details of construction—aligning all of those mundane, ordinary and challenging matters right in front of us with the highest ideals of life, yoga practice and who we most truly are.

Questions to Consider and Write About

1. What is your intention in practicing yoga, or in creating a spiritual practice?
2. Why explore the idea of building a temple of the body?
3. What does building a temple of the body mean to you?
4. In beginning such a process, what do you hope for?
5. What do you long for?
6. What is your highest aim and how can you relate it to being free from what currently holds you back or makes you feel unworthy, alone or incapable?
7. In what ways, if any, do you feel unworthy, separated from or incapable of having such a high intention?

two

The Highest First

> *Our highest intention is to see and experience the universal everywhere and in everything, within and without, in the full range of diversity.*
>
> —John Friend

I call this first principle of building a temple of the body "Put the Highest First." This idea echoes teachings from several esoteric traditions. It is an attitude and a context more than a physical technique, and might be seen more as a state of being than a state of doing. Yogi Ramsuratkumar called the Highest "My Father." Many traditions call it God, others refer to Supreme Consciousness, grace, Spirit or the Divine. Regardless of what word or words we use as labels (and in this book I will use these terms interchangeably), "putting the Highest first" means cultivating a state of remembrance: That all our personal efforts are gestures of affirmation to help us experience ourselves as part of a larger spiritual flow.

The philosophies that inform my yoga practice state that everything is supreme consciousness. "There is nothing that is not Supreme Consciousness."[1] These elegant philosophies describe one sublime energy that goes through a series of transformations, in a stepping-down-type process, until that one energy has taken on a multiplicity of forms. Much like a rainbow, in which one light has different wavelengths along a spectrum of color, this one energy, this one light, is at the source of all that is. The immanent world of form or manifestation is seen as a result of the different wavelengths of the one light that create different colors. In these traditions, God does not create the universe. In these philosophies, God *becomes* the universe. There is nothing other than God.

With this uncompromisingly non-dual outlook, we see that no part of creation is essentially separate from the whole or the Highest. And yet I am not suggesting, nor do the traditions that inform this viewpoint suggest, that all things are equal. Or put another way, "It is all One" does not mean "Everything is the same." We must cultivate discernment and maturity as we align our practices with these ideas. While all things are the Highest in an ultimate sense and essentially auspicious at a fundamental level, in the world of relativity with its many levels of being, not all aspects of the Highest are the same. For instance, some actions cause harm to others. Some actions diminish beauty. Certain actions bring us closer to our ideals. Some choices diminish our capacity to serve one another. There are ethical, moral and even legal domains to consider.

Ideally, the actions that we take in our sadhana and the skills we cultivate in our practices will help us to cultivate the ability to put the Highest first more effectively in all that we are and all that we do. Practice is one means by which we remember our truest self, a means by which we put the Highest first. Just as building a temple of the body is as much an intention as it is an outcome of practice, putting the Highest first is both the means as well as the goal of our yoga. And while practice is absolutely essential, in other words while our efforts are absolutely required, the first principle reminds us that they are only part of the formula. Our efforts must be in relationship to the flow of the Highest; our practices must be guided by and dedicated to serving its flow.

Essentially, we practice by joining our efforts with the Highest. A verse in a scriptural text called *The Kularnava Tantra* states that, "By entering the current of the Divine Shakti's descent into heart, the true disciple becomes capable of receiving Grace."

Professor Douglas Brooks expounds:

> Here in one of the most elegant and subtle statements about yogic practice made anywhere, we are offered a powerful and practical insight: the sincere practitioner of yoga, the true disciple, gains access to the Divine's own creative energy by entering into the Divine's presence which has descended into his or her own heart. By touching the current of Divine Grace flowing through our bodies, minds and hearts, we gain access to an entirely new, awakened and joyous experience of life. What is required of the yogin is to open the heart in order to experience this freely given gift of grace, which naturally flows through our being. To open our hearts to this grace is to experience directly that Divine presence.(2)

So, we are told that our efforts will be met by grace. When we align ourselves optimally, we will become capable; we will be *made able* to experience the flow of grace as the gift of capacity from the Highest. We cannot do "it" alone, nor are we intended to.

Enlightenment or Not

Anyone who has studied yoga over a period of time knows that not all traditions of yoga see the task at hand in this same way. For instance, the Yoga Sutras of Patanjali, as they are classically translated and utilized, teach that yoga is a means of culturing oneself so that the consciousness, or the *citta* (in Sanskrit), is stilled, allowing the stainless purity of the soul to be reflected. That state of stillness in the mind that is cultivated through meditation is called *samadhi* and is considered by Patanjali to be the goal of yoga.

My experience is that putting the Highest first may or may not have anything to do with "stilling the mind" in the way that these earlier schools of yoga suggest. Putting the Highest first seems to have a flavor that is, at times, entirely different than seeking enlightenment and/or samadhi as defined by Patanjali in the Yoga Sutras. While not unrelated to classical yogic aims, putting the Highest first is also its own paradigm of spiritual life—as much about discipleship as it is about mastery, and about participation as much as it is about renunciation.

My teacher Lee Lozowick's website contains only one sentence: "If you're looking for enlightenment, go somewhere else . . . and while you're at it, grow up." Lee has quite an acerbic wit, so for years I thought he was kidding and making fun of us "seekers" with that statement. One day it dawned on me that he just might be serious. I realized that he, as a teacher, might not be offering his students enlightenment *at all*. He, and therefore we as his students, might be up to something else entirely. Instead of being schooled in samadhi or enlightenment, I began to consider that we are being trained in the art of devotion, the yoga of discipleship and the joy of conscious living.

As Lee Lozowick's student, I have learned about discipline, managing my mind, serving others, accepting life *as it is* and the necessity of hard work, sacrifice and dedication. I have experienced states of exaltation and of deep contentment. The number of synchronicities relative to my prayers have led me to believe in the miraculous, but have also established within me a level of trust I never knew outside of his company. Honestly, he has given very few if any talks on samadhi. And I cannot remember one mention of "how to still the mind" so that no thought waves remain.

True Happiness

According to Kirsti, a devotee of Yogi Ramsuratkumar's, one day the Beggar was "nearly rolling with laughter, his hands over his face and slapping his knee." A person nearby, observing this hilarity, remarked, "You certainly are a happy man!"

The Beggar turned to the man and, his eyes sparkling, said, "If there is love in a man's heart the whole world will be beautiful." —Regina Sara Ryan, *Only God, A Biography of Yogi Ramsuratkumar*, 625.

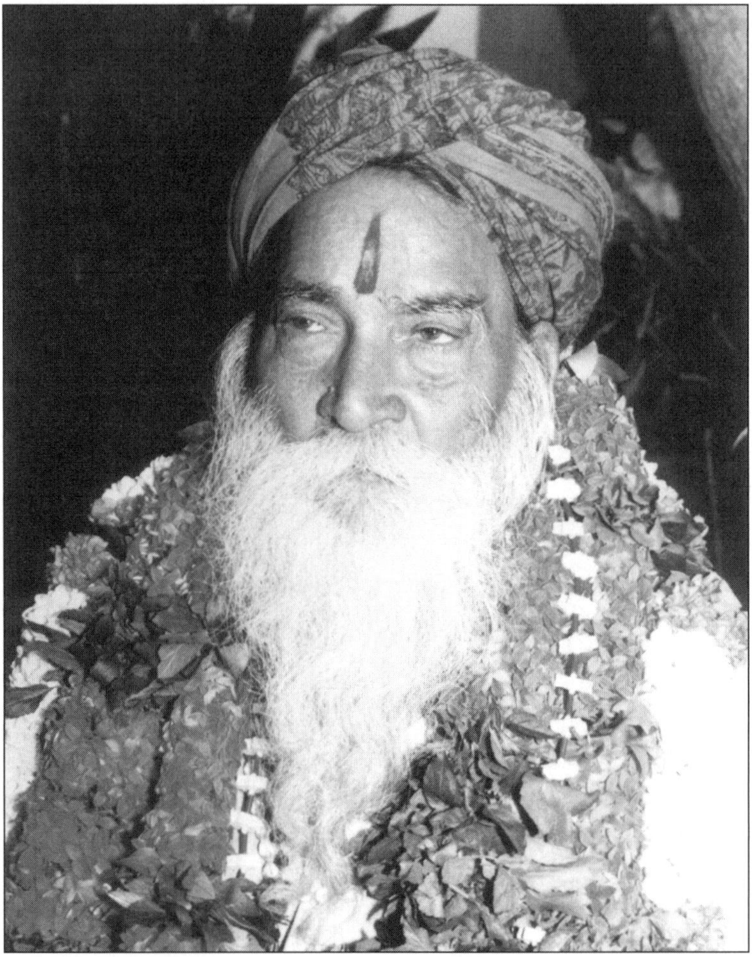

Yogi Ramsuratkumar

Therefore, this is not a how-to book about samadhi as it is classically defined. It is a manual of practice aimed at pointing us to a life of service, devotion, and discipleship that is at the foundation of the temple-building project because "yoga . . . is a discipleship to the flow of God's love and will." (3) This book is aimed at helping us to align with a source of inspiration that resides in the innermost chambers of our heart, and with developing the skills and virtues necessary to skillfully navigate the currents of this flow.

A Different Aim, A Different Mood

I have found that establishing putting the Highest first as a yogic aim, context or intention, as opposed to samadhi, yields a different mood for practice. I had the opportunity to study asana in India with several master-teachers who practice yoga with "stilling the mind" as their aim. Over the course of a two-hour class one teacher described the details of the upright posture that was required for effective pranayama and meditation. She described the necessity of training oneself to manage all of these details to set the proper stage so that the prana would flow optimally in the body, thus yielding the desired effect, the experience of samadhi. At one point, she looked at us, all of whom did not seem to be getting it and said, "God is not going to come to your meditation just because you ask him to!"

I knew what she was getting at. For instance, simply saying to yourself, "I have put the Highest first," is a reasonably simple affirmation to recite, while the true spirit of actually doing it is not so simplistic. The yogic path is an arduous process, engaged by only a few, realized by even fewer. This teacher was trying to impress upon us the exacting nature of the path and all that is required of the practitioner. I appreciate that.

But it also struck me as a great example of different yogic aims, different guiding principles for practice. While this teacher believed that God would not visit someone just because that person asked God to, my personal experience is different. Truth be told, God *has* come to me for no other discernable reason than my simple request. God did not necessarily come to me in the form of still *citta*, but most definitely in the forms of lifesaving interventions, answered prayers, insight, clarity, friendship, opportunities to serve, to grow and to choose a life that lies beyond my habits and personal preferences.

Along similar lines, I have a student who went to a yoga class in a method that emphasizes stilling the mind. The teacher interviewed her when she arrived to make sure that the level of class was appropriate. At the conclusion of the interview, the teacher looked at my student and said, "Well I hope you are here ready to listen, to learn and to work hard. Otherwise it is never going to happen for you."

When my student told me this story I was shocked to hear that a teacher would say this to a student she had never met before. But it was my student's response to the teacher that was truly inspiring. She told me that her first thought was, "It has *already* happened for me. It happened for me in my very first class." My student went on to tell me that she knew her alignment wasn't 100-percent perfect, that she knew she had lots to learn and that she was far from "done," but the *yoga had already happened*. She had already aligned with something decidedly spiritual and she had already been met. Her longings had led her to yoga. Yoga had opened her heart and given her a taste for more. Put another way, her efforts had joined the Highest, her efforts had aligned her with grace and she glimpsed something profound within herself—within life itself.

These stories highlight what to me is the most distinguishing feature of our endeavor to build a temple of the body—the recognition that the Highest is the essential guiding principle of all that we do and all that we seek. With this ideal guiding us, we enter into a more expansive understanding of samadhi than "still citta" or "the highest form of meditation." The expanded understanding of samadhi that we find in a grace-oriented practice is based on the meaning of the root words themselves. *Sam-* means "together" or "integrated" and *-dha* means "to place" or "to put." So in a certain way, samadhi means "place together." Expanding on the etymological definition we might see samadhi in a new light, as that state where we put all parts of ourselves "together in the same place." Instead of samadhi being a state where there are no fluctuations in the thought waves, or instead of seeing it only as a state of meditation, for the purposes of building a temple of the body we can look at it as that state where all of our thoughts and actions are brought together toward the singular aim of putting the Highest first in all that we are and all that we do, as a discipleship to the Highest itself. Instead of stilling the thoughts, we are joining them together as an act of devotional offering to the flow of the Supreme. In this way we are bringing our whole self together in yoga. And we are seeing ourselves as together with everything in the world—as essentially the same as the things and the people around us.

I am very clear that Patanjali, in the Yoga Sutras, was talking about samadhi as a state of meditation, and I am not attempting to rewrite Patanjali's yoga sutras here! What I am talking about here is by no means a classical definition. But this consideration can have practical applications to our spiritual practice, nonetheless.

Thou Art That

Putting the Highest first is also the recognition that, essentially, we *already are* that which we seek. This yoga is not a perfecting process to get somewhere, but a process of recognizing who we already are. And while putting the Highest first may sound mystical, big, and even hard to fathom, putting the Highest first is also quite practical, immediate and accessible to each of us. The longing to find our true nature, and the longing to find sanctuary and meaning, and the longing to genuinely serve something greater than ourselves are not such foreign or abstract feelings. I believe these feelings exist inside the heart of each sincere practitioner who sets foot on the path of yoga. These longings fuel our efforts and deliver us to the foundational principle of building a temple of the body where we recognize that the alignment we are seeking is only possible with a connection to something beyond the personal domain.

Putting the Highest first establishes the largest possible context for our endeavors. Rather than simply practicing for physical reasons, putting the Highest first places our physical motivations within a context of spiritual unfolding. So, whether or not it is likely that on any given day of asana practice we will experience samadhi or pierce the nature of reality, we dedicate our efforts in asana to a larger purpose. In the words of yoga master B.K.S. Iyengar, "We begin how we wish to proceed."(4) We aim high. We begin by assuming that, not only is it possible, but that it has already happened because *we already are* essentially part of the flow, rather than by assuming that we are not ever going to "make it." In putting the Highest first we give voice to the deeper urges that live within us, to those longings to align ourselves deeply to the truth that lives in each of us; and everything around us.

In order to build a temple of the body we must remind ourselves that there are deeper forces than our individual personalities that inform the world; that deeper forces than our ideas and our ideals are at play; and that these forces are beyond what our modern day scientific paradigm has yet proven. We might call this remembrance a "spiritual context," although my personal opinion is that the word "spiritual" is over-used and misunderstood and fast on its way to becoming completely useless to actually describe anything. (But let's use it anyway! Why not?) A spiritual context means that the questions you ask may include things like, "How can I be happy?" and "How can I learn to love myself?" but they also include considerations of service, sacrifice, discipline, discernment and so forth. We must learn to make distinctions between the human heart with its hopes, wishes and dreams, and our essential spiritual heart, which may demand that we sacrifice our human heart's impulses from time to time. In other words, we must see that the fundamental spiritual heart is at the deepest essence of the human heart and it's desires. We must reconcile, or bring together, these aspects of ourselves through our yoga practices.

Bold Step Forward

Engaging the principles and practices of yoga is, in many ways, a bold step forward. In choosing a life of practice, in choosing to build a temple of the body, we are placing ourselves in a stream of service and devotion to something larger than our individual whims that will demand that we continually grow, change and refine ourselves to become more and more fit to the task. It is a bold proposition to leave a life of creature comfort and personal preference in order to build a temple of the body. We will need to discard outmoded thoughts and beliefs, overcome our resistance, and time and again choose to align our actions with the highest ideals of the heart in order to create momentum toward our deepest aims.

Most modern schools of hatha yoga don't require a specific set of practices in order to participate. For instance, it is rare that anyone is required to be a vegetarian or to be monogamous if they want to come to yoga class and be part of the community. But, as we will see in future chapters, most systems of yoga do offer a thorough set of ethical guidelines based on traditional principles of *yama* and *niyama*. Practice and ethics are not seen as rules to follow based solely on some external authority, but are, instead, guidelines that bring us into integrity with our intrinsic goodness and help us to "glorify the Highest and to align ourselves with that which is life-enhancing, beautiful and auspicious."(5) The principle of glorifying the Highest is ideally at the heart of our personal choices as we build a temple of the body.

The intense, sincere desire to glorify the Highest, the fundamental beauty of life, and to align ourselves with what is life-enhancing, beautiful and auspicious is at the foundation of our motivation to engage any discipline. Think about why we might want to stop smoking, stop abusing alcohol, stop overeating or stop acting out in anger. Certainly the first level of the answer might be that we want to avoid the pain that these things are causing us. And, if we look a little deeper, we will see that some aspect of ourselves knows that we *are fundamentally and essentially worthy* of a better quality of life than these painful outcomes of destructive behavior.

If we are following a spiritual teacher's recommendations or a given tradition's guidelines, another reason that we might engage such discipline is that we choose to be obedient. As we explore the deeper levels of obedience, then, we may recognize that obedience to a true spiritual authority is nothing other than obedience to that part of ourselves that is intrinsically authoritative because it is through that part of ourselves that we are already essentially linked to the source of our spirituality. It is this deep part of us, the part that is already connected to the Highest, that we can strengthen by living a life of dignity and practice.

As we build a life that glorifies the Highest, a life that is in relationship to what is essentially beautiful, many times we find that we outgrow old patterns. We often find that there is less room for the destructive behaviors, pessimistic outlooks, unkind thoughts and words because the life-affirming choices have what one of my mentors calls "the majority vote."

Majority Vote

Getting to the place where our life-affirming choices have the "majority vote" in our lives seems, in my experience, to be a result of three things: grace, effort and renunciation.

Grace: This idea of grace playing a vital role in our ability to practice is an underlying idea of 12-Step recovery as well. In my experience, addiction was doing something I did not want to be doing, over and over again. For years I would wake up and promise myself that I would not binge or purge that day. And, as the day progressed, the urge to act out would arise and I would try my best to abstain. I would try very hard, and then, inevitably, I just would succumb to the desire. The binging and purging was a compulsion.

Most recovering alcoholics will say similar things about their recovery from alcohol. Many people have spent years "swearing off" and promising themselves and others they would change before they ever got sober. They literally *did not want* to be drinking and yet they were. This is a very common experience. In my case, I did not want to be overeating and yet I was. To be compelled to behave in a way that one does not want to be behaving is a basic perspective on addiction. And, we should keep in mind that addictions can exist on the level of our mental attitudes and self-talk as well as in our gross behaviors.

Initially, the only thing that made a difference in my addictive behaviors was prayer. I begged God to remove from me the compulsion to overeat so that my power of choice could be restored. In the grip of the compulsion, I had no ability to choose. I *had* chosen "not to," sworn a solemn oath to myself to abstain, and yet time and again, I still went through with the addictive behavior.

I am aware that this idea of "no ability to choose" is a controversial one. After all, the ideas of choice, free-will, compulsion, obsession and addiction confront some of our deepest notions of personhood, and rub against some of our most existential beliefs. I share this perspective not to convince anyone, but simply to explain my direct experience that, at certain stages of the game, we cannot change or employ a practice through force of will alone. Many times there are influences at play beyond our conscious, rational minds that are both working for and against us. Therefore, sometimes, we will need the power of Grace.

Effort and Renunciation: The second and third influences in the process of establishing ourselves in practice and/or making changes in our behavior seem to be opposite ideals. They are, in fact, quite complimentary as they create a balance of positive and negative energies. Balancing the negative and positive aspects of sadhana corresponds to two qualities—*abhyasa* and *vairagya*—as outlined by Patanjali in the Yoga Sutras. Abhyasa is our longstanding efforts, done with reverence and without interruption. [This principle will be discussed in greater depth in Chapter 3.] Abhyasa is the positive acts of practice—like eating a healthy diet, practicing asana, meditation and pranayama.

Vairagya asks us to cultivate a freedom from passion and from attachment to the outcomes of our effort. Vairagya refers as well to a conscious renunciation of those things that do not serve our lives as practitioners. These two aspects of sadhana complement one another. As we practice, the light is strengthened and we are able to let go of those behavior and attitudes that have kept us in the dark. We begin to experience small tastes of being aligned with and joined in our heart's aim. And as we glimpse that integrated state, it inspires us to practice. We are inspired to renounce what doesn't serve us, and consequently we glimpse more unity and integrity. *Like that.*

Practice is a result of eradicating (that is, renouncing) the negative, and growing (efforting) the positive within the field of the Highest. We will need to do both renouncing and efforting. We can focus on and become aware of the "untruths" in our lives and study the ways our negative patterns are blocking us from aligning with our true nature, and make sincere efforts to renounce these negatives. And, we can study the truths that are within us and build on them, making sincere gestures to grow the positive.

In asana practice for instance, when someone in my class has a hurt shoulder, one of the things I do is examine their alignment and look for the imbalances that might be contributing to their pain. After looking for the good and seeing the auspicious and true flow of energy in their body, I study the "untruth." I look at what is blocking the flow or what is in the way of optimal. But in order to evaluate what is blocking the flow, I first have to know *what optimal alignment* for the shoulder actually is. I need to know the "truth" of the shoulder. Then, I teach the student how to apply principles of alignment to bring their body out of misalignment and "into the flow of the Highest." Yoga then becomes a process of awakening to the truth, moving from the untruth to the truth and of aligning with the Divine. In order for healing to take place, students must dedicate themselves to creating a set of actions that will line them up optimally, thus allowing the body's innate healing power to arise.

In general, rather than only examining what is dysfunctional, we align with the Highest and apply our "efforts" to moving toward optimal (abhyasa). In moving toward optimal, the dysfunctional is minimized (vairagya) and then replaced altogether. Many times what must be "renounced" in these situations is over-effort, pushing, unrealistic expectations for the body and the tendency to ignore the signals of pain and injury. Other times it is not doing enough or not feeling like we are capable to do at all.

The same principles of effort and renunciation apply in matters of the heart and emotions. In psychological work, it can be helpful to inventory our patterns. It is useful to understand the beliefs that contribute to our positive and negative personality traits. We may benefit from examining how these traits relate to our childhood upbringing and adapted coping strategies. We will certainly have to renounce certain behaviors and tendencies that we find are working against ourselves, but, at a certain point, we must apply ourselves to growing the positive traits more than trying to rid ourselves of the negative. Darkness cannot exist in the presence of light. Instead of continually examining the darkness, we light candles of new attitudes and behaviors until we have created a circumstance within us where the light has replaced the darkness.

These three aspects of practice—grace, effort and renunciation—create the ground upon which we become disciplined, mature practitioners. Whether the area of our foundation that need helps is our diet, our exercise regime or our pursuit of study, we will encounter and rely on the magic of grace, the power of renunciation and the necessity of positive action. With these principles at our foundation we can engage a life of practice not as some set of imposed rules but as something we *want to do* out of loving respect and a natural and sincere desire to glorify the Highest.

When Yogi Ramsuratkumar built his temple he did not say, "I want to build a temple as a creative expression that I will enjoy and have fun at." He said, "I want to build this temple so that it will provide sanctuary and blessings for others." He clearly built the temple as a means to serve others. By the same token, we can certainly use yoga to cultivate our own happiness. But we can also cultivate ourselves and build a temple of the body so that through our happiness, through our physical stamina, we are able to serve others, serve life, and therefore serve the flow of the Highest.

Questions to Consider and Write About

1. What does it mean to put the Highest first?
2. What does it mean *to you* to put the Highest first?
3. How do you recognize when you are aligned with the Highest?
4. In what ways have you experienced the Highest in your life?
5. Do you believe you are worthy of the Highest? Do you act as if you are?
6. What do you consider to be the highest aim of your heart? Of your spiritual heart? How might you reconcile those two?

three

PRACTICE

I believe that we learn by practice. Whether it means to learn to dance by practicing dancing, or to learn to live by practicing living, the principles are the same. In each, it is the performance of a dedicated, precise set of acts, physical or intellectual, from which comes shape of achievement, the sense of one's being, the satisfaction of spirit. One becomes in some area an athlete of God. Practice means to perform over and over again, in the face of all obstacles, some act of vision, of faith, of desire.

—Martha Graham

Abhyasa (practice) is a dedicated, unswerving, constant, and vigilant search into a chosen subject pursued against all odds in the face of repeated failures, for indefinitely long periods of time.

—B.K.S. Iyengar

Deciding to build a temple of the body is not a decision to simply make your body healthier, although in the process you might get healthier. Building a temple of the body is not a diet, although in the process you might change your eating habits. (Of course, you might not.) Building a temple of the body is not a program of self-improvement, a set of precise instructions, a promise of happiness or a guarantee that you will get stronger, thinner or more attractive. Building a temple of the body is, in fact, a call to a life of spiritual practice.

In most hatha yoga circles of which I am a part, practice usually means doing asana. For the purposes of building a temple of the body, practice implies a way of life that aligns us with the Highest. It includes, but is not limited to: the things we eat and the things we do not eat; the way we talk to ourselves and the way we talk to others; the way we manage our minds as well as our behavior; the way we breathe; the way we conduct ourselves in relationships of all kinds; and the remembering of the reason behind our various choices. Practice encompasses learning from mistakes, as well as our response to our failures and shortcomings along the way. Practice also includes more formalized rituals like prayer, asana, meditation, mantra recitation, study and contemplative writing.

In the Yoga Sutras of Patanjali, he suggests that there are three criteria for something to be considered a practice: 1. the action (or actions) must be done constantly, without interruption, 2. the action (or actions) must be done over a long period of time, and 3. the action (or actions) must be done with reverence.

Think about it. Each of us does many things repeatedly over long periods of time. Take brushing your teeth before bed, as an example. Just the fact that we brush our teeth every day (i.e., constantly and without interruption) and that we have brushed them every day since we were children (i.e., over a long period of time) does not make brushing our teeth a *practice*. Why? Because there is no reverence or conscious devotion present. However, it is possible to take the mundane act of oral hygiene and transform it into practice by establishing a higher context for our actions. For instance, we might stop taking our teeth for granted and recognize that it is actually a gift to have teeth. We might cultivate the idea that keeping our teeth clean and free of damaging plaque and tartar is an act of gratitude for the gift we have been given. And, in that remembrance, devotion arises. If that devotion can be brought to bear upon the simple act of brushing our teeth then, *voila*, we have a practice.

In the same way that brushing our teeth became a gesture of devotion, building a temple of the body invites us to engage our entire lives as practice. Building a temple of the body will require more of us than simply committing a few hours a week to practicing asana, no matter how great the asana is or how much we love it. Building a temple of the body will require that we build a life of practice.

I once heard a yoga teacher give a talk on this topic. He sternly told the group that while most of us have deep and sincere revelations when we practice asana and pranayama, most of the insight and change that we think we are experiencing is merely cosmetic. He suggested that this was the truth because we have failed to change at the level of our unconscious tendencies. He said that by the time we have put away our yoga mats most of us have returned to what is the equivalent of being "sub-par humans"; we have begun to criticize ourselves, to judge one another, to gossip, to ruminate, to worry and live as though the practice we just said was life-changing had never happened.

I do not think this teacher was indicting us to make anyone feel bad. I do not think he was discounting the reality of the insight gleaned from practice, or negating the sincerity of anyone's desire for personal transformation. I think he was pointing out that insight and profound opening experiences must be met with constant practice over a long time in order to take root. Those *aha* moments must be put to practice, brought to life and sustained in every aspect of our lives or else they are, as he suggested, merely cosmetic changes.

Ideally, the time we spend practicing asana, particularly if that asana practice is infused with actions that physicalize our deepest intentions, helping us to embody virtue, will actually help us to build a life off the mat that is integrated with the life we have on the mat. In my first book, *Yoga From the Inside Out,* I described a process of making peace with my body that I engaged after many years of self-destructive acting out. While asana practice assisted my process of healing, asana was and continues to be only one piece of the puzzle. Changing a lifetime of habits takes a lot of effort, a lot of time and tremendous devotion. It takes practice.

The word *abhyasa* is the Sanskrit term for practice. Abhyasa is made up of two parts: *abhi* which means "repeatedly and intensely facing the goal" and *-asa* which means "to sit or abide" (as in the familiar word asana). The word abhyasa itself teaches us what practice really is and what is required of us to become practitioners. We must be *seated in*, we must *reside in*, the repetitious and intense process of facing our goal. Whether the goal you are facing is to be a better parent, to lose weight, to forgive yourself or someone else, to build a temple of the body or simply to establish a daily asana regime, rest assured that you are going to meet challenges and obstacles along the way. If you met no obstacles you would not be in the domain of practice. If these behaviors came easily, we would be talking about recreation, not practice.

A Life of Practice

At least once a week a student will share with me the difficulty she or he is having in establishing a personal asana practice. Typically, these students are not beginners. These are experienced students who love to practice asana, who come to class regularly, and who, in most cases, are quite proficient; yet they are having trouble establishing a personal practice outside of class. For most people, motivation is not the problem. They are motivated. They really want to practice. For most, loving and enjoying the yoga is not the obstacle. Truly, most of these people love and enjoy yoga. Something else is the obstacle. There is a weak "muscle" hidden somewhere that must be revealed and strengthened in order to succeed and face the goal.

I think the weak muscle working against many people in establishing themselves in any practice is twofold. The first part is having unrealistic expectations. Most people I talk to expect it to be easier to practice than it actually is. For some reason, and I am not saying that this is conscious on anyone's part, many of us think that because we have motivation it should be easy, when in fact it is nothing of the sort. Even to practice asana for thirty minutes, one needs to prioritize the time, carve out a space, have the knowledge and the confidence to begin, the materials necessary, someone to watch the children, and the ability to turn off the TV, put off the chores, or not look at the email. One will face seemingly endless distractions just to put out a sticky mat at home and practice asana. Why do we think it should be easy? Thinking it will be easy does not prepare us at all for what is actually required.

Let's go back to the teeth-brushing example. As easy as it seemed a few paragraphs ago to make oral hygiene into a spiritual practice, think realistically about how difficult it would be to actually do it. Every single time you brush your teeth you will need to be mindful, devotional and aware of the higher context you want the act to embody for you. Even when you are late, even when the kids are screaming and even when you are in a fight with your mate, you will need to remember. Even remembering to remember will be a challenge many days. If something we are already doing, like brushing teeth, is hard to keep established in the context of practice, think about how hard it will be to practice something that requires a new set of behaviors!

Additionally, many times we expect that once we decide to practice our progress will be swift, when in all likelihood it may be tediously slow. As a personal example, I first went to therapy for bulimia when I was sixteen. My psychiatrist asked me how I would like my relationship with food and my body to be. I remember describing to her that I would like to feel good about my body. I wanted to be able to go swimming and not feel so self-conscious about my body that I couldn't even enjoy the activity. I told her that I wanted to be able to start eating when I was hungry and to stop when I was full. Those were my goals then. In all honesty, while lots of progress was made along the way (and certainly lots of mistakes), I was probably thirty-six when I realized that, on most days, I ate when I was hungry and I stopped when I was full. (And that I loved to go swimming!) Twenty years later I was established in my goal. So in yoga, we are talking about a timeframe that confronts and challenges even the most patient among us.

There is a famous yoga school where they have ongoing asana and ongoing pranayama classes. After five years of asana studies students are eligible to enroll in the pranayama classes. For the first year of pranayama classes, students are not allowed to practice the breath techniques, they are instructed to simply practice *savasana* (corpse pose, relaxation pose). The theory of this approach is that one should not practice pranayama until they can relax properly. After a year of relaxation training, students begin to learn pranayama. They are then considered beginners for ten years. On a similar note, I had a teacher who used to say that no matter what poses you can perform, you are a beginner for the first five years of your practice.

I tell these stories to illustrate that the yoga timetable is something in which very few of us have any experience. Most of us would have a hard time being a beginner for five, much less for ten, years. More often than not, we try to advance as quickly as possible, thus attempting to fit yoga into our paradigm of rapid progress, rather than adjusting our expectations to fit with yoga's paradigm of progress and practice (intensely facing the goal, with reverence, over a long period of time, in the face of all odds). Just as bodies can take a long time to change, longstanding beliefs and feelings often change even more slowly. Truly, one must cultivate realistic expectations.

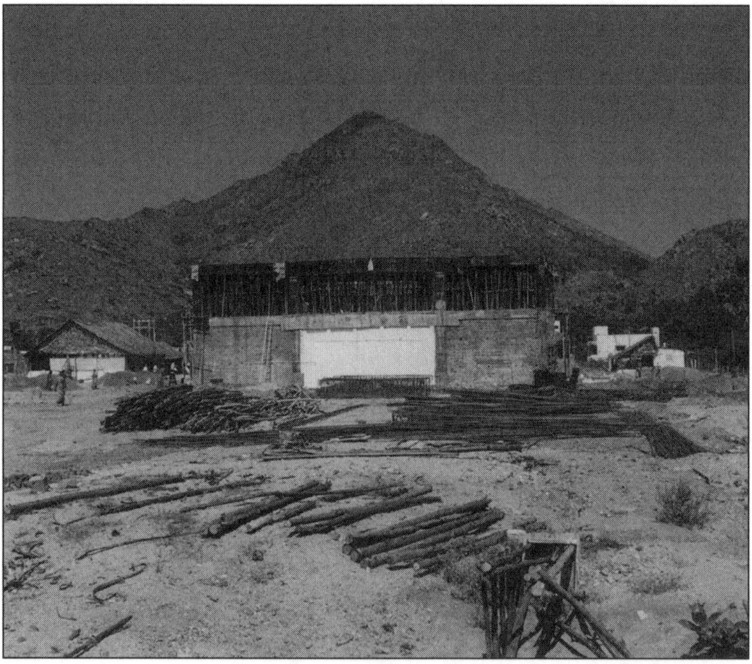

The sacred mountain, Arunachala, presides over all; in this photo, the early work on the Temple of Yogi Ramsuratkumar, Tiruvannamalai, South India, 1994.

Practice as Love

The second aspect of the "weak muscle" I mentioned is that many people fail to see practice as a loving act and to see themselves as worthy of such love. The longer I practice yoga, the more obvious it becomes to me that what sustains me in practice, and what has helped me implement any positive change over time, is love. Truly, eating a healthy diet is an act of love. Practicing intelligent asana that honors and challenges my limits is an act of love. Sitting still and quiet in meditation is an act of great love in a culture of stress, rushing and distraction. Cultivating compassion, discernment and the ability to see beauty are some of the nicest things I could do for myself.

I find it shocking that in our culture we often celebrate with self-destruction. How many times have you been following a healthy eating regime only to "reward yourself" with something that is unhealthy or downright poisonous? How many people celebrate their joy of the New Year with so much alcohol that its entire first day is spent hung over? Consciously or unconsciously, we frame a life of practice—which is basically a life that, through skillfully made and sustained choices, embodies our intention to recognize ourselves as part of the flow of the Divine—as something that we need to rebel against. Why is it that we do not see such rebellion as a rebellion against all that is good and true within us?

The simple answer is that on some level we do not see practice clearly. We see it as an imposition of values rather than an alignment with what is already dignified within us. We are trained to try to make ourselves better rather than to see ourselves as good and then act accordingly. My belief is that the more we practice as an act of love, the more our intrinsic goodness is revealed. The more we are established in our direct experience of this goodness, the easier it becomes to choose behaviors that support and uphold our realization and to live in alignment with the flow of the Highest.

This process of learning to live in alignment with the Highest is a process of refining ourselves through the loving acts of spiritual practice or sadhana. Practice can become something other than a set of imposed rules and admonitions from an external authority based on some ideal of the perfect yogi we are supposed to become. Practice can become a set of attitudes and actions—of efforts that we bring to grace—that align us with the remembrance that who we most truly are, as a part of the flow of the Highest, is dignified, noble and essentially good.

Questions to Consider and Write About

1. Why practice?
2. Do you typically practice or try to create changes from a place of love or from a place of criticism? Why do you think this is?
3. In what aspects of your life might you cultivate more loving discipline?
4. What happens for you when you meet obstacles in your practice?

four

Intrinsic Goodness—Looking for the Good

It is not just an arbitrary idea that the world is good, but it is good because we can experience its goodness. We can experience our world as healthy and straightforward, direct and real, because our basic nature is to go along with the goodness of the situation. The human potential for intelligence and dignity is attuned to experiencing the brilliance of the bright blue sky, the freshness of green fields and the beauty of the trees and mountains. We have an actual connection to reality that can wake us up and make us feel basically, fundamentally good.

—Chögyam Trungpa Rinpoche

Finally, brethren, whatever is true, whatever is right, whatever is pure, whatever is lovely, whatever is of good repute, if there is any excellence and if anything worthy of praise, dwell on these things.

—Philippians 4:8

The fundamental context of building a temple of the body is that life is essentially good. Life, as the expression of the Highest, as the Divine in form in the relative world, shares its basic nature with that of the Divine. Therefore, the fundamental attributes of the Divine at the absolute level are the attributes of creation, of life itself, of each one of us. Those who study yoga philosophy will learn different words, concepts and means by which to express this idea of intrinsic goodness, but they all express what is essentially a basic idea: if the energy of which we are made is essentially good, then we too are essentially good.

While scriptural study can help build an intellectual matrix through which we can encounter and examine these ideas, the direct experience of intrinsic goodness can be found only through practice and with the help of grace. We cannot study our way to experiencing our intrinsic goodness. We must assert its truth and look for it in every moment. To be very clear, I am not discounting the importance of scriptural study. On the contrary, I love scriptural study and philosophical inquiry. But while certain philosophical constructs and explanations can be found in books, the direct experience of these ideas is certainly more valuable and can only be found when our participation joins our contemplation.

Skillful Means

As yoga practitioners interested in building a temple of the body, we must chose to participate with life in specific ways. This type of specific participation according to yogic principles is called skillful means. Skillful means assists us in making distinctions between what is life-enhancing and what is destructive, between what serves the aims of our heart and what takes us away from them. One of the skillful means that we must develop is the ability to see the good even in the midst of chaos, turbulence and fear. This is part of what we mentioned earlier as having a spiritual context.

Having a spiritual context or looking for the good is not a simple practice. I personally struggled with this teaching for many years. I still do. It is not my first impulse to see what is good or to remember that my optimal context is larger than my opinions, ideas and preferences. Initially, my first layer of resistance to intrinsic goodness and "looking for the good" came from my real experience and those of people I worked with—things were *not* always so good! We did horrible things to ourselves and to one another. Repeatedly, even when we knew better.

As my understanding matured, I gained clarity into the different domains of reality that this philosophy assumes. Absolute goodness is on an ultimate level, which is a different domain from the relative world of pain and sorrow. This goodness is said to exist beyond the duality of good and bad. This made sense to me. I could move forward. The next level of resistance I worked through was that, on some level, looking for the good seemed kind of phony to me. I couldn't shake the feeling that it was an overlay of a good script or some kind of new-age affirmation exercise.

Even though I had my doubts about looking for the good, I still practiced my teacher's suggestions. In the yoga classes I taught, I made it a point to look for what was good, beautiful and true in my students. And the process of looking for and speaking to what was good began to change me profoundly. I began to see that this practice of looking for the good was training me to be more at peace, more content, and was helping me to recognize the tremendous amount of support I had in my life. Simply put, I was getting happier. It wasn't that my life circumstances changed. *I* changed. I was able to see how good everything actually was. Fundamental nature was revealed. Absolutely nothing changed externally, and yet, everything was somehow better.

Also, in the midst of my personal process, the yoga communities in Arizona of which I was a part, were struck by two violent tragedies. In Tucson, Anusara Yoga instructor Emmade was murdered in his home. A few weeks after Emmade's death, Anusara Yoga teacher Desiree Rumbaugh's son, Brandon, was murdered. In less than one month, our community had been affected by violent, random crimes that were about as far from good as you could get. And yet, I watched myself and I watched the people directly affected by these losses cling to the teaching of intrinsic goodness and it did not fail them. It was not easy—people's understanding and naiveté was confronted, but the teaching did not fail. Each person I knew, myself included, took the teaching, funneled it through his or her own experience and came to an understanding of what it meant for them. Desiree shared with me a little about her personal process:

> Someone just gave me a "Life is Good" t-shirt this weekend. My first one ever. I am glad they waited until now to give me one. I couldn't have worn it one day earlier. I do agree that life is good and now I can say it, but up until now, I couldn't just stop there. I would have had to say that life is good and bad . . . sometimes life is bad. Really bad.
>
> In order for my mind and heart to finally begin to accept the untimely departure of my son from this earth, I had to wrap my head around the concept that each soul has its own pre-determined path and that we are all extremely independent from each other. That type of thinking is what saves me from bitterness or from feeling like a victim.
>
> The problem with that thinking is that it makes me want to steer clear of any kind of "intertwining"

with another . . . Now, would I have been like this anyway? Maybe. But now, even more so. A separate soul on a separate path should have a lot of privacy and I feel like I need to figure things out on my own and not depend on anyone in particular.

Having said this . . . I can now see the "It's all good" philosophy beginning to work for me again. Because for Brandon, it is *all good* that he is off to his next chapter now. For me, it is sad if I think about what I missed out on by not having him here, but for him, I can only imagine that he was finished and that he is really happy now.

I have received abundant blessings in this life and also my share of some heavy-duty pain. I think most people do. When I meet people who haven't had the heavy-duty pain yet, I don't feel jealous. I just feel neutral. I wouldn't wish this on anyone. When I meet those who know this kind of pain, there is a kinship between us. There is a bond of understanding that you have to have experienced to understand.

Somewhere along the line I feel I must have agreed to some kind of deal where I would lose my son in this lifetime. Many people have. God knows what else I agreed to. I guess I will find out eventually. What I have learned from this is to live only in the moment. While it is true that I have plans for the next two years all laid out, I do have to live into them one day at a time.

I have less fear than I might have for having gone through this . . . and yet I do fear the possibility of losing my other child, Jessica. But, I have thought through that, and from here it looks like a complete identity shift would be an option. For instance, I think I would move to India, change my name and work in

> an orphanage. I didn't realize how closely attached I was to my identity as a mother. The ones who have it rough are those people who lose their only child or all their children.
>
> And yet . . . bitterness is a very sad option to choose and to stick with. Perhaps it is actually more work to remain bitter than to just let go. I have simply chosen to let go and let God . . . as trite as that may sound. It seems like my best choice.(1)

In Desiree's contemplations one can see the themes I have noted. She has had to move through layers of accepting *what is* in its relative good and bad (even really bad) manifestations to come to a more expansive view of goodness. It is not an easy task, and yet we see in her sharing the quality of practice and choice she has embraced relative to her ideals and philosophy. Obviously, she was dealt a circumstance that confronts trite "it's all good" platitudes. She had to go much deeper.

We all have to keep digging deeper to bring this philosophy to life. While this teaching is simple on the surface, and upon first glance is quite reassuring, in the midst of life's upheavals it is actually easier to say "this is good" and "this is not good," or "this is Divine" and "this is definitely not Divine" than it is to embrace the perspective of "it is all God and therefore intrinsically good."

Facing the Truth

Looking for the good is not a way, nor should it be used as a way, to avoid the necessary suffering that comes along with being alive. Looking for the good does not ask us to hold in our grief, ignore our anger, mask our frustrations and run away from what is true for us in the human domain. Emotional honesty and maturity is actually an important part of how we learn to make the distinctions necessary to be effective practitioners. Remorse, regret, grief and the sincere disappointment we feel when we have failed our best intentions are all important fuel for our sadhana. Many times, we cannot see what is good no matter how much we look for it until we have processed these kinds of difficult emotions honestly. We must see things clearly, as they are.

Seeing things as they are, however, is a multifaceted process because reality is multidimensional. Often, several things are true at the same time, and some seem to conflict. The apparent conflict stems from the fact that we are in a process of *both* being and becoming. There is a truth that is consistent with our state of being—it boils down to the basic ideas that: there is a flow of the Divine, of the Highest; the flow is intrinsically good; we are part of that flow, and therefore we are intrinsically good. This is certainly "what is."

In the process of becoming, however, we may not be aware of this being-level truth. In our process of becoming, for instance, we may feel "less-than." We may feel unworthy, separate, alone or incapable. These feelings are true and real as well, within their own domain. They also are "what is."

Looking for the good is seeing "what is" on an essential level, at the level of being. Looking for the good, as a practice, is choosing to look for the reality that is true at a level that is deeper than personality and circumstance. It is the assertion of our spiritual context, not an overlay or fluffy affirmation process.

My student Stephen has struggled with this aspect of yoga philosophy in his own sadhana. He once shared with me how important it is to him to see "what is." We had an ongoing email conversation about yoga philosophy and personal practice. After discussing "it's all good" and "accepting what is" and the way that they relate in our lives, he wrote:

> The "seeing what is" thing is so important. They call that phenomenology in Western philosophy. We need to simply observe phenomenon rather than constructing and superimposing conceptualizations that are largely divorced from the context they are seeking to frame and understand. That being said, I do have an experience of the good. And it is sweet and full of *shri*. And I can connect in my own way to the . . . ethos but it does take some translating . . . [(2)]

In my opinion, that process of "translating" goes on for most of us. This translating is simply the way that we make sense and relate to the teaching as our own. And making the teaching your own is of the utmost importance.

My philosophy teacher Carlos Pomeda talks about three levels of inquiry we need in order to effectively engage the study of philosophy. The first level asks the question "What?" What does the teaching actually say? What does it actually mean?" What did it mean in its original context and time period? The second level of inquiry asks "So what?" What does it mean to me? Given this 2000-year-old teaching of samadhi, given this teaching about looking for the good, what does that mean to me, here in the second decade of the twenty-first century, in central Texas with my particular set of neuroses, opinions and talents? How do I translate this idea to me and my life? The third level of inquiry involves the question of "how." How do I practice? How do I bring this context and what it means to me alive through practice? Like we talked about earlier, how do I not only learn how to read the recipe but learn to cook and get to eat and enjoy the meal?[(3)]

I loved Stephen's comments because they highlighted how, even in the midst of the mind's problems with the words and the ideas, Stephen had the direct experience of goodness. He had eaten the meal. And even though the heart has enjoyed the meal, the mind may always be finding fault with the recipe! This common dynamic between the heart and the mind is why our contemplative practices like meditation and journal writing are essential for our progress on the Path. We must become intimately acquainted with our mind's voices and learn to distinguish them from our heart's voices. We must recognize the "part" of ourselves who is eating the meal, the part who is still pondering the menu, and the part who won't even sit down at the table.

Once again, integrating these ideals is a practice for most of us, and progress is made slowly over time. There may always be voices within the mind that have a problem with looking for the good, practicing yoga and with anything that conflicts with our habitual behavior. After all, we are raised in a world that prioritizes comfort and personal freedom. We are indoctrinated into a dualistic view of the world, in which certain things are good and others are evil. We are used to black and white lists of right and wrong. Typically, we are not trained to see things as they are. Many of us are not naturally skilled in seeing the essential goodness when pain is what is most prevalent. But as we practice, as the Divine reveals to us its goodness, our heart begins to experience a different level of truth and we become more and more established in our spiritual context.

All Is God

My teacher Lee Lozowick often says that, as devotees, we need to see everything in life that happens as the blessing of Yogi Ramsuratkumar. Sickness, health, fame, fortune, financial ruin—all are to be regarded as his blessing. In our Western Baul tradition we regard Yogi Ramsuratkumar as the literal embodiment of God. Therefore, all things are him and because his nature is always blessing, all things are his blessing. As we mature, we learn that not all blessings are easy to take, not all circumstances are equally pleasant, and perhaps they *become* his blessing not because the content of the occurrence was "good" but because they yielded within us a movement toward spiritual life—an ultimately good outcome.

Keeping Context: The Task of the Project Manager

Yogi Ramsuratkumar's ashram manager and supervisor of the temple building project was a devotee named Mani. Mani had lived for close to fifty years with little interest in religion, spiritual life or gurus. Over a short period of time, however, Mani was brought into the intimate company of Yogi Ramsuratkumar, serving him directly in several different capacities. Even though his devotion and service were nearly impeccable, longtime devotees of Yogi Ramsuratkumar were uncomfortable that a "newcomer" was elevated to such a position of authority, responsibility and personal access to the guru. At times, the longtime devotees were so threatened by Mani's status that they complained to Yogi Ramsuratkumar that Mani wasn't fit for the job . . . unqualified for the position. After all, they said, Mani had a history of socializing; he had been a businessman, he ate meat, etc. How, they asked, could he be an ashram manager?

Mani tells many of these stories in his memoir, *A Man and His Master* (Hohm Press, 2003). He refers also to his hurt feelings, and his frustrations with ashram politics, but most importantly, he shares Yogi

Ramsuratkumar's instructions to him regarding these difficulties. Yogi Ramsuratkumar told him, "It is all Father's Blessing."

I do not think that Yogi Ramsuratkumar was insensitive toward Mani's feelings, but I do think that his job as the guru was to keep Mani established in context, in remembering that while all of these things were hurtful personally, the reason he was even at risk of being criticized was because he had the opportunity to help Yogi Ramsuratkumar build a temple. The circumstance of being able to serve in that way was a blessing, so therefore, everything that came with it—all difficulty and all challenge—was part of that blessing. Truly, it was all good.

Questions to Consider and Write About

1. Do you believe in intrinsic goodness?
2. In what circumstances, if any, might you find it impossible to believe in intrinsic goodness?
3. Is it harder for you to see your goodness or to see other people's? Why do you think that is?
4. Is there a time when looking for the good would not be a good idea?
5. In what ways do these ideas affect the way you see yourself?
6. What is good about you? What is good about someone you do not like?
7. What is good about your yoga or spiritual practice?

five

The Body

The mystical, the truly miraculous, is here, and absolutely nowhere else. The doorway is now, not when the presumed obstacle of the body is out of the way. In fact, most people have no idea how literal that description is. We have this illusion that we need to get the body "out of the way" so we can do "real work" or so we can be undisturbed and unhindered by the confusion of emotions and organic urges and desires. But such a circumstance is literally "out of the Way." The Way, that is the spiritual path, the practice of sadhana or of awakening, the Work, is about using what the body makes accessible and possible in all its radiant glory, in all its profuse confusion, with all its three-centered mess, as the gift of God, as the very—in fact, the only—opportunity to advance along the Great Process of Divine Evolution. The body, as it is, inclusive of all its elements, levels, gross and subtle, chemical, energetic and "spiritual" is entirely who we are. The body is the Body of Work, the Body of Practice. The body is the Way, and not the "way out" but the Way directly to the heart and soul of God.

—Lee Lozowick

Although I will be using the temple of the body as a guiding metaphor as I write, it is important to understand that the body I am referring to is a body that includes, but is not limited to, the physical body. According to the Vedic yogic traditions, each of us actually has many "bodies." These bodies are sometimes referred to as the *kosas* or the sheaths (coverings) of the essential self. These sheaths are often pictured like nesting Russian dolls surrounding the *atman*, or the soul. The innermost layer is known as the "bliss sheath," followed by the "sheath of wisdom," the "sheath of the mind," the "sheath of the vital force" and the outermost layer is called the "food sheath" because it—our physical body—is built from the food that we consume. Even from this very brief and generalized foray into yogic anatomy, we begin to see that we are multilayered, multidimensional creatures, and that as yoga practitioners our idea of the body is quite inclusive.

In order to build a temple of the body we must take into account the different layers of our being. We must build our temple in such a way that the construction is sound at all levels. If all aspects of ourselves are working together toward the revelation of the essential self, then we would truly be aligned with our deepest intentions. The good news is that change on one level affects change on another. Just as our bodies might get sick during times of emotional stress, the opposite is also true. If we bring the gross body into physical balance, many times the mind and the emotions become more balanced as well.

Kaya Sadhana and Tantra

Kaya sadhana means the cultivation of the body as a means for spiritual transformation. This type of sadhana points us to a stream of yoga philosophies and practices that has come to be known as tantra. I say "has come to be known as tantra" because when these schools of practice arose, they did not refer to themselves as tantric schools per se.

"Tantra" is an academic designation used to talk about yoga schools that have certain commonalities. While scholars point out that the roots of tantric philosophy can be found as early as 500 BCE in various rites and rituals across India, tantra as a school of yoga flourished in India between the ninth and fourteenth centuries of the common era (CE). Yoga scholar Georg Feuerstein states that "historically . . . *tantra* denotes a particular style or genre of spiritual teachings that affirm the continuity between spirit and matter." Feuerstein explains:

> *Tantra* is a Sanskrit word that, like the term yoga, has many distinct but basically related meanings. At the most mundane level, it denotes "web" or "woof." It derives from the verbal root *tan* meaning "to expand". . . This root also yields the word *tantu* (thread or cord). Whereas a thread is something that is extensive, a web suggests expansion. *Tantra* can also stand for "system," "ritual," "doctrine" or "compendium." According to esoteric explanations, *tantra* is that which expands *jnana*, which can mean either "knowledge" or "wisdom."
>
> But *tantra* is also the "expansive," all-encompassing Reality revealed by wisdom. As such it stands for "continuum," the seamless whole that comprises both transcendence and immanence, Reality and reality, Being and becoming, Consciousness and mental consciousness, Infinity and finitude, Spirit and matter, Transcendence and immanence, or in Sanskrit terminology, nirvana and samsara . . .[1]

We see in tantra, and in the schools that are categorized as such, a radical evolution in philosophy and practice. No longer was the spirit seen as separate from matter in the way that the classical yoga of Patanjali suggested—that *puruhsa* (spirit) and *prakriti* (matter) were distinctly different. No longer was this world of form seen as an illusion based upon our ignorance (*avidya*) of reality, as the Advaita Vedanta schools of the time posited (*advaita* literally means not-two, non-dual). Here, in these revolutionary schools of tantra, yoga practices were based on the idea that the nature of the Divine was twofold—transcendent *and* immanent. In the tantra schools, the yogis were interested in the "continuum" of consciousness that informed everything.(2)

This radical philosophy yielded some interesting developments in the way yoga was practiced. The body and the world of form were no longer seen as essentially at odds with a life of the spirit. Instead, the body and the manifested world were regarded as expressions of the spirit, and therefore seen as essentially Divine. This is what is meant by a non-dual perspective. One of the distinctions between the non-dual perspective characteristic of many schools of tantra and the non-dual perspective characteristic of many Advaita Vedanta schools is that tantra sees the manifest world as essentially real, whereas vedanta regards the world as essentially illusory.

This distinction about the essential nature of the world creates a different "yogic task" for the practitioner. If the yogi sees the fundamental existential dilemma as one of misperception, of mistaking the illusory for the real, then one's sadhana must be aimed at seeing clearly, at overcoming this mistaken perception. If, however, the yogi's view is that the immanent world is as real as the spiritual world, one's guiding precepts and, therefore, resulting practices, change quite profoundly. In this view our essential yogic dilemma is one of a contraction of spirit, and therefore our practices are aimed at expanding our consciousness to see our true, expanded state of being.

This change, also known as "the tantric turn," is summarized quite nicely in a few verses from the Kularnava Tantra scripture, translated by Dr. Stephen Phillips. In this short excerpt the prevailing yoga paradigm of transcendence and world-denial is being compared to the tantric paradigm of immanence and world-affirmation.

> (2.23) If a yogin, then not at all could one enjoy the world. If enjoying the world, then not at all would one be skilled in yoga. The Kaula (a particular Tantric path) is of the nature of enjoyment and yoga. Therefore, dear one, it is universal.
> (2.24) If one follows the Dharma of the Kaula, O Queen of the Family, enjoyment becomes yoga immediately, misbehavior becomes art, and all of life is liberation.[3]

To the sincere tantric practitioner, yoga, instead of being a path of denial, renunciation and transcendence, becomes a path of embodiment where skillful participation in the world of form is the means by which a yogi directly experiences the nature of the Divine. To be clear, while the text clearly states that enjoyment is not a problem and can, in fact, be its own yogic mechanism, this is no way implies the free-for-all of indulgence that many people unconsciously equate with enjoyment.

For example, is it truly enjoyment to drink so much alcohol that you regret things you say, fall down, and are sick the following day? Is it truly enjoyment to eat in such a way that over a period of time your body carries so much extra weight that your health is compromised? Is it really enjoying chocolate when you eat the whole box without even noticing what you are doing? Is it really enjoyable to smoke and ingest a noxious fume that is proven to cause cancer and emphysema and to weaken your immune system? Is it actually enjoyable to gossip in hurtful ways? Are these indulgences true enjoyment? Absolutely not.

Again and again, the mature practitioner must learn to make distinctions about what serves the flow of the Highest, what creates beauty, and what has value over the long term. These passages cited above, from the Kularnava Tantra, are most likely written for the practitioner who is living a disciplined, sane life of yogic practice. Rather than an excuse to "do whatever you want and call it tantra," these inspiring verses point us to a possibility of practice that uses everything—every circumstance, thought, emotion and mistake or seeming misbehavior in an unrelenting, uncompromising affirmation and exploration of the ever-present nature of grace.

Great Possibility

This tantric path of radical affirmation has exciting possibilities for those of us interested in building a temple of the body; of establishing a life of practice that is, at its essence, a joyful alignment with the Highest. The ramifications of such a philosophy funnel all the way down to how each of us regards his or her own life circumstances, choices and relationship with the body.

Instead of looking at the body and the world as *other than* the path, we see them as Divine, as useful and necessary to our awakening. And awakening, according to these traditions, is not an acquired state but a state of waking up from a dream of being separate from God, recognizing that we already *are* in a state of grace. Ultimately, this philosophy underscores an empowering way to live because it places the responsibility of our spiritual life squarely in our hands. We do not need anything other than what we have and what we are in order to practice yoga. We do not need fancy equipment. We do not need to escape to the mountain top. We simply need to cultivate the skills necessary to make use of all that we are, and all that we have been given, in order to expand our consciousness and wake up from the dream of sleep.

Yogi Ramsuratkumar's temple was built to be a blessing force. The finished building was the literal manifestation of Yogi Ramsuratkumar's state of being, which was constantly blessing. Therefore, everything involved in this temple project was important, essential and sacred—each nail, every brick, each piece of rebar, each person's effort was necessary.

Just as Yogi Ramsuratkumar's temple was the manifestation of his state of being, so too is our temple of the body and every aspect of ourselves important, essential and sacred. Just as Yogi Ramsuratkumar's life's work was embedded in the brick sand mortar of his temple, so too can our life's work be to build of ourselves, of our body in its totality, a temple that will embody and glorify the Divine with which we are essentially One.

Questions to Consider and Write About

1. What does "the tantric turn" mean to you?
2. How does a life of enjoyment blend with one of spiritual practice?
3. What areas of your life are tipping the scale toward indulgence? Toward denial, abstinence, or asceticism?
4. What areas of your life are probably "just fine," but still you feel guilty about them?
5. Are there things about your personality or life that may seem like obstacles or negative that you can also see as blessings of the Divine in some ways?

six

Asking the Right Questions

I would like to beg you dear Sir, as well as I can, to have patience with everything unresolved in your heart and to try to love the questions themselves as if they were locked rooms or books written in a very foreign language. Don't search for the answers, which could not be given to you now, because you would not be able to live them. And the point is to live everything. Live the questions now. Perhaps then, someday far in the future, you will gradually, without even noticing it, live your way into the answer.

—Rainer Maria Rilke,
Letters to a Young Poet, 1903

Yogi Ramsuratkumar knew clearly why he wanted to build his temple. Although his inspiration and intention were set, still he needed land, building plans, permits. He needed a project supervisor and people for work crews before he could commence building. Similarly, those of us who are building a temple of the body, if we desire a successful endeavor, will benefit from planning and from clarifying our agenda. For instance, we will need assistance; we will need to know what the lay of the land is before we get going. We can ask questions in three basic domains to guide our planning: why, how and what?

1) *Why* do I want to build this temple? Why is my heart longing for this?
2) *How* am I going to build it? Do I have the know-how, so to speak? and
3) *What* do I need to do? What actions will I need to take?

Even with a cursory glance at these questions, we see that the heart has to have a reason (why), the mind needs to know how (how) and the body is going to need to act to bring the vision into manifestation (what).

The Problem with Answers

Werner Erhard, the founder of est, is famous for saying that "Understanding is the booby prize." On a similar note, yoga master B.K.S. Iyengar says that, "Yoga is not an intellectual game, it is a sharing of real experience." Both of these teachers are pointing to the same idea, I believe, reminding us that simply understanding something is not the same as experiencing the truth firsthand.

Like many of us, when I am too quick to satisfy my intellect, I often truncate the process of real self inquiry. As soon as my mind figures something out or has an answer, I stop actively exploring the idea. My mind actually convinces me that I know something, even though my behaviors and my heart may not be demonstrating that knowledge.

For instance, you have heard, "The body is a temple and therefore we should treat it with love and respect." Obviously, this statement rings a bell of truth and you may think to yourself, "Yes, that is true. That explains it exactly! I should take better care of myself." But then in the next hour, or over the next few days, you overeat, you over-consume alcohol, you smoke cigarettes, you ignore your body's signals of pain in asana practice, you drink too much caffeine, you fail to sleep adequately, you eat foods that are full of chemicals and proven carcinogens, and so on. While the mind knew the answer of why you should take care of yourself, the questioning of how to bring that truth to life had ended before the knowledge was integrated into reliable, disciplined action. That deeper inquiry had stopped, and therefore the higher perspective was not realized.

So, while we can see that the intellect is satisfied by answers, the heart is only satisfied by soul searching, trial and error, and by the oftentimes painstaking process of refining oneself. We must be careful not to allow the intellect's initial satisfaction with answers to seduce us into living only in the fascinating realm of thoughts and ideas. We must continue exploring the questions of the heart, even if the questioning process grows uncomfortable as it asks us to confront unexplored regions within ourselves, or to change our behaviors that no longer serve our movement toward truth.

As we practice, as we build a temple of the body, we must learn to ask meaningful, useful questions about our endeavors. Best is that we do not ask things like, "Why is it so hard?" Instead, we might ask, "How can I keep at the forefront of my mind why this hard work is necessary?" Best that we do not ask, "How can I make this easier?" when we might instead ask, "Is this effort worth it?" Answers are a function of the questions we ask. If we ask questions about how to grow as practitioners, we will get answers that assist us in deepening our sadhana. If we ask questions about how to be more comfortable along the way, those are the answers we will receive. If we ask how might my life and my actions support the creation of a temple of the body, a place of sanctuary, refuge and service, we will more likely experience the potentially transformational gestures of our sadhana.

Satisfying and Gratifying

My yoga teacher John Friend makes a powerful distinction between what is satisfying and what is gratifying. *Gratification*, he says, is usually found in the short term, provides a payoff in immediate pleasure, and is often at the expense of our heart's intention. For instance, the second helping of food, the snooze button, the catty thoughtless remark, our overspending, and any attempt at shortcutting are usually driven by that part of us that is seeking gratification. While these choices may feel good in the moment, over time they can compromise our yogic aim.

Satisfaction, on the other hand, is to be found in those endeavors that require patience, determination, tenacity and perseverance. This satisfaction comes only from living in those questions of the heart, from cultivating our strengths, and from facing our resistances honestly and reliably. Satisfaction is the result of having the discrimination and ability to delay gratification long enough to allow something more meaningful to be built in its place. "We learn," John Friend writes, "to differentiate between fulfillment of our spiritual desires vs. gratification of our physical desires. All of our short-term physical desires and wants are put into the larger spiritual context of how their gratification may or may not serve our long term spiritual desires and intentions."[(1)]

This same principle of discernment applies to asking questions. We can learn to ask questions from the domain of satisfaction—questions from the heart, about practice, about deeper truths—rather than questions based in gratification, namely, questions motivated by self-concern and egoistic preservation. In our inquiries we can learn to go deeper than curiosity and deeper than being right. We really *can* learn to tell the difference between a head answer that may easily satisfy the intellect with immediate answers or explanations and a heart answer that keeps us passionately exploring. We really *can* build the capacity to choose the heart's journey over the life of the mass culture and our personality habits. We really *can* build of ourselves a great temple. And we can build it like any building—with a plan, with help, from the ground up. Then we can furnish it, decorate it and live there.

Patience Is Crucial

> Something Bhagwan had said started to take root in me—He had emphasized the need for me to have patience. He said, "Patience is crucial for Mani to endure the trials and adversities inherent in doing the work of this Beggar's Father. To be patient means to suffer something that hinders or haunts us, something that disturbs and hurts us, and still retain self-composure." Patience could elevate and strengthen our character. His teaching was not a philosophy to be learned or practiced; his teachings had to be experienced and then embodied in daily life. —Mani, *A Man and His Master*, 107.

The Sadhana of Questions and Answers

With many of the deeper questions of the heart, the answers lie not in arriving at any one right answer but in cultivating the capacity "to live the question," as Rilke encouraged his young poet friend. Learning to ask the right questions is only one part of the process. We have to engage the answering process skillfully as well. I consider this questioning and answering process as a vital aspect of sadhana or practice.

Any idea presented in this book is meant to be practiced, not achieved in the sense of completing something and then putting it away on a shelf. The extent to which you actually take these ideas to heart, work with them, explore them, filter them through your direct experience, is the extent to which they will actually help you. Put another way, the extent that each one of us lives the question—in our hearts, words, thoughts and actions—of "How can I build of myself a great temple that serves my highest potential?" that building process will be meaningful and effective and connected to our highest intention, our samkalpa.

Questions to Consider and Write About

1. What does it mean to you to "live the question"?
2. What do you do to avoid "living the question"?
3. How do you cope with questions that cannot be answered simply?
4. What are some of your important questions? What is the head answer? What is the heart answer?

seven

Attention

Prana is the energy that drives life, the power that animates the body, enlivens the mind, spurs the soul. Prana is life's inspiration, its foundation, its tenacity; it is the sure hand on the tiller, the wise voice of good counsel, the urge to health and harmony that craves to turn our bodies into havens where we can take shelter from the storms of the hectic modern world. Prana is at work at every instant in every cell of every living organism, seeking ever to deliver us from disease and confirm us in health, but only in those few people who are genetically fated to be healthy does prana automatically regulate its momentum. The rest of us must learn how to cultivate our prana.

—Robert Svoboda

Yogi Ramsuratkumar was intimately involved throughout the process of building the temple at the Yogi Ramsuratkumar Ashram.

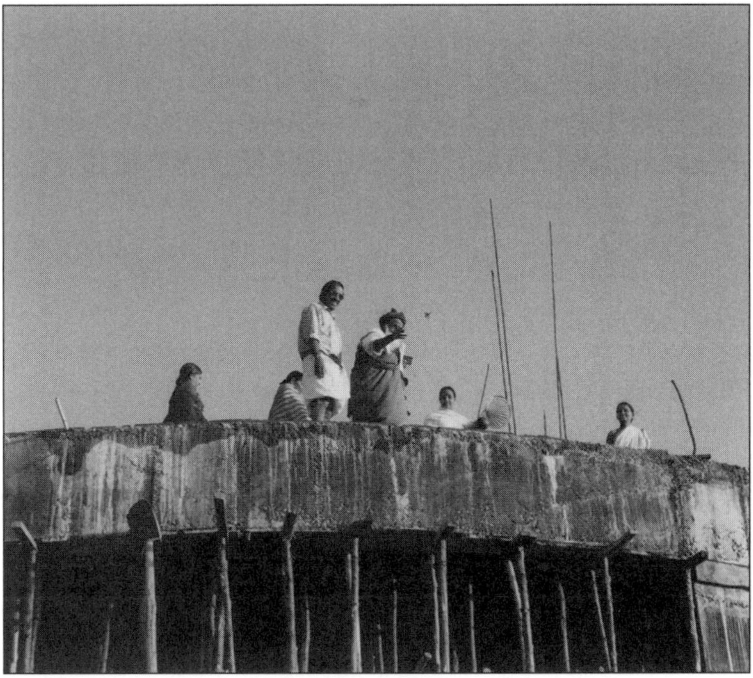

Yogi Ramsuratkumar tosses a flower from the roof of the temple construction. Mani stands at his side. 1994.

Mani, the building project manager, writes:

> He blessed every aspect and detail of the building of His Ashram—the land by walking barefoot, the trees by touching them, and the workers by His continuous blessing and His precious and radiant presence.
>
> He would visit every part of the Ashram to see the work, but not just to look at it to see the progress. He would examine different places and spaces so closely, with such particular attention, as if He was filling them with something powerful. He would gaze at empty spaces where a building was going to be made. He fused raw materials with life-force, walking around or

> sitting on piles of bricks, bundles of steel bars, and lorry-loads of sand. It always brings tears to my eyes when I think about His attention and care in every detail, looking at the raw materials, staring at the space in the air where the dome would be fabricated. It was as if He was building the dome Himself in another dimension with His intention, and we were following His intention with crude materials to make it visible to our mortal eyes. We would have to use sand and minerals and water and energy to transform the air into the shape he already formed with his gaze.(1)

When I first contemplated this aspect of Yogi Ramsuratkumar's story in reference to building a temple of the body, I immediately saw the similarities to asana practice. In asana we cultivate the ability to pay attention on multiple levels—to our heart's intention, to the placement of our bodies in space, to the actions required in any posture to maintain alignment, to our breath, etc. The more advanced the yoga practitioners become, the more details of alignment there are to which they attend.

In my experience, alignment-oriented methods of yoga are misunderstood by those practitioners of yoga who do not concern themselves with biomechanics, classical forms and the pursuit of optimal alignment. These methods of yoga often say that the alignment methods do not focus enough on the deeper purposes of the practice, or enough on the breath; or that we are too perfectionistic; or that teachers have to talk too much in order to guide students into such intricate alignment. And while all those observations may contain some element of accuracy, they are far from the truth in terms of the true invitation that skillful alignment instructions provide the practitioner.

Alignment in asana practice is not divorced from deeper meaning, as some critics suggest. Alignment is actually the means by which we bring the larger meaning and context of practice alive. Every asana practice can begin with a contemplation about how the practice can serve to bring each practitioner into greater alignment with, and into a deeper experience of the heart—the heart of who we truly are, the heart of the Highest that is at the core, or heart of everything in life.

This heart, with which we seek to align ourselves, is not the heart of emotions that is concerned with personal happiness, and the like. It is the spiritual heart, one's essential nature. This spiritual heart is regarded as the gateway to the experience of Divinity or of grace itself. This heart with its highest ideals becomes the guiding, organizing principle for all our efforts and gestures, from the way we place our feet to the way that we breathe.

Prana follows attention.

—Yogic concept, quoted by Robert Svoboda

Because alignment exists on so many levels, it becomes a means by which we cultivate our attention and therefore our prana. Because prana, our life force, moves toward that to which we pay attention, attention becomes a valuable tool in anything we are trying to accomplish. It gives us momentum.

When we endeavor to build a temple of the body, we must bring a fullness of attention to our building project, as if we, like Yogi Ramsuratkumar, were infusing the very bricks with our attention and blessings, so that we have the necessary momentum to accomplish our task. By training ourselves in asana to pay attention to the details of life on the mat, we are simultaneously training ourselves to pay attention to the details of life off the mat. Building a temple of the body takes place in several domains—in formal practices like asana and pranayama, in the mundane aspects of our daily life, and in the advanced yoga of life's trials and tribulations.

Truth be told, our attention will always be placed *somewhere*. The invitation of yoga, the invitation to build a temple of the body, is an invitation to consciously choose what you will pay attention to, and to develop the skills required to sustain your focus and the momentum necessary to keep moving in the optimal direction. Rather than allowing ourselves to be swept away by shallow cultural imperatives and unconscious motivations, yoga teaches us to stay focused on what most deeply serves us, the highest ideals of the heart and of the Highest itself.

Questions to Consider and Write About

1. In what direction is your overall life momentum taking you?
2. In what direction would you like your momentum to take you?
3. What behaviors create negative momentum in your life?
4. What behaviors are creating positive momentum?
5. What do you place your attention on negatively that has inadvertently aligned you with something other than your highest ideals or deepest truths?

PART II

LAYING THE FOUNDATION

Having established an optimal context for our endeavor, this part explores the foundational practices that concretize our ideals and create the solid ground floor upon which to build our work.

eight

Adhikara

On February 22, Bhagwan asked me if I would begin my work for Him by marking the building plan on the leveled ground of the Ashram. He showed me the drawings for the Ashram plan, which He said was "approved by Father."
—Mani, *A Man and His Master*

In asana practice the foundation of a pose is any place that touches the ground. In standing poses our feet and sometimes one or two hands touch the ground. In supine positions, the back of the body is the foundation. Inverted postures, like headstand, have the head as part of their foundation. And so on. To lay the foundation is to optimally place that part of the pose that meets the earth. Optimal placement is relative to each pose, and because the poses vary in form so does the optimal placement. Additionally, optimal placement increases the possibility for the Highest to expand within our posture.

For instance, if you step your feet wide and keep your feet facing straight ahead, the pose is called *prasarita padasana*. If you turn your feet to the right, the pose is now called *parsva prasarita padasana*. Regardless of which way your feet are pointed, however, there are some general principles that apply to every pose. For instance, no matter what part of the body comprises the foundation, it has what we call "four corners," and there is a specific methodology to placing these four corners so that the foundation of our posture is level, solid and of sound construction.

Because our practice is one of embodiment, of deep involvement in and the radical affirmation of life itself, the way that we as practitioners touch the ground is of utmost importance. If the Highest is to be engaged here and now, on the earth, in and through the body, then our foundation must be solid in order to be prepared for the work to come. The way we set our foundation should reflect our intention to align with the Highest. If, for instance, we want to practice the pose *trikonasana* (triangle pose), but we do not place our feet correctly, we might risk injury to our knees. If we want to practice *pranayama*, but we do not have the foundational knowledge of how to proceed, we might harm our nervous system either through over stimulation or suppression. If we want to serve others, but we are not grounded enough to see what is needed in the given situation, our help might actually be harmful to the other person or to ourselves. If we wish to build of ourselves and of our lives a temple of the body, but the basics of our general conduct is at odds with the Path, our lack of foundation will thwart our efforts before we can even break ground and start to build.

Ready Ready Ready

The yoga traditions have always placed great emphasis on having a good foundation and on preparedness. In Sanskrit this preparedness is called *adhikara*. Sometimes translated to mean "studentship," the word adhikara is made up of two parts. *Adhi*- means "ready" and *-kara* means "to make." Adhikara, then, can be understood as "making oneself ready, to clear the bar, to prepare oneself or to be prepared" for practice.

Adhikara, our preparation and preparedness, is the aspect of the temple-building process over which we have dominion. After all, we cannot determine exactly *how* our temple will turn out, or be used. We cannot determine in advance exactly how any project will turn out. What we can do is prepare ourselves along certain lines. We can take the leap of faith that is required but, after a certain point, the process belongs to the Highest and we will need to relinquish some of our personal ideas, opinions and preferences.

Keeping Faith

> Bhagwan gave us the opportunity to understand certain things—in the case of the bore well, we had our doubts about the prospect of getting water—it's like having faith or not. The machinery strikes the earth, tunneling into the darkness of it, not knowing when water will be reached. It was a valuable lesson to have happened so early in the construction work. According to the water table information we would strike water at two hundred feet. When that didn't happen we began to doubt the selection of the site by the diviner and Bhagwan. It was our own doubtful ideas that would not work. We were complaining that the well diggers would not reach water because the facts were that we should have by two hundred feet.—Mani, *A Man and His Master*, 161.

The age-old adage of "work without attachment to results" comes from this idea of adhikara. We, after all, cannot be responsible for the fruit of our actions, but we can be responsible for how we prepare ourselves and for how much we apply ourselves to the efforts required.

Making oneself ready to practice yoga has many levels, just like our intention exists on many levels. Think about all that goes into to just getting to yoga class. In order to make yourself ready on Monday night, for instance, you have to leave work on time, drive through rush-hour traffic, arrange for childcare, make dinner ahead of time or buy it for your family on the way home. You must confront your mental fatigue, your end-of-the-day hunger and your desire to just relax. Adhikara, being ready, for yoga practice is no small task!

On deeper levels, adhikara implies that at the foundation of our sadhana is a sense of resolve. We have decided to practice. We have decided to put ourselves in a stream of aligning with the Highest. Adhikara is that state of readiness within ourselves that has the necessary faith and tenacity to see the project through, even when we are met with obstacles.

Adhikara is not built quickly or easily, neither is a temple of the body. Yogi Ramsuratkumar's temple was not erected overnight either. Like many aspects of yoga, adhikara is both a means of practice and practice's end result. As much as we make ourselves ready to practice, our practice also makes us ready to live fully, to face our unique challenges with honesty and integrity. What is the reward of adhikara, of practice, if not the ability to keep practicing! The only way we can get strong enough to overcome the obstacles to practice is to face them, confront our weaknesses, and with the help of the Highest, to grow the necessary muscles to keep practicing.

The Need for Faith

Because of the challenges inherent in our task, we must remember that our building project has a uniquely high purpose, and that our plans need to ultimately be aligned with the highest ideals of awakening and expanding joy. We need faith to appreciate that, because of the sanctity of our purpose, our efforts will be met with help from the Highest.

At the beginning of construction on Yogi Ramsuratkumar's temple, for example, there was a significant shortage of materials. In order to break ground, they first needed to measure and mark off the locations of the buildings but they did not have adequate measuring tools. When faced with the obstacle of a tool shortage, Mani, the project manager, could have sat down, complained that he did not have the necessary equipment, and taken the rest of the day off. Instead, he was so committed to his task that he used whatever he could find to get the job done. Yogi Ramsuratkumar, seeing his resolve and effort, came to his aid. The aid came first in a tangible way—Yogi Ramsuratkumar himself held the rope and helped Mani with the measuring—and secondly in a more subtle way, as Yogi Ramsuratkumar kept this measuring rope with him, literally around his neck, for the remainder of the project, as a covenant between master and devotee.

Mani's *Adhikara*—Effort Meeting Grace

There were obstacles but I was not going to let these difficulties prevent me from doing what I had been asked to do by Yogi Ramsuratkumar. Somehow I came upon a length of rope and started to measure and mark the area. Bhagwan was there at that time. He came up to me and asked, "What will Mani do with that rope?" I explained the purpose to Him.

He said, "Mani, will you allow this beggar to help you? This beggar would like to hold this rope at one end. Mani can measure from the other end of the rope."

Such was the beginning of my work for Him. He was right there assisting me, seeing that the makeshift tools were accepted and blessed. We measured the area according to the plan with the rope I had found lying somewhere. After the work, Bhagwan called me and asked, "Does Mani need this particular rope?"

"I can manage with some other rope also, Bhagwan," I said.

"Mani should permit this beggar to keep the rope with him."

I said yes immediately. He made the rope like a garland around His neck. He was keeping that same rope for so many years after. To me that rope signified that no obstacle would come between Him and the completion of His Ashram. . . .

When Bhagwan assigns some work, He has already finished that work. In the material world, we are simply projected as His Instruments to make the work manifest. We have no business to think about feasibility; we should be like an athlete getting ready to run a race. We need to have the utmost concentration and be empty of all conflicting thoughts. As we begin to run this race, we should remember that while we are running toward the goal, He will take us to the finishing point. There is no doubt about this. We must have impeccable commitment and absolute faith in Him.—Mani, *A Man and His Master*, 101-102, 97.

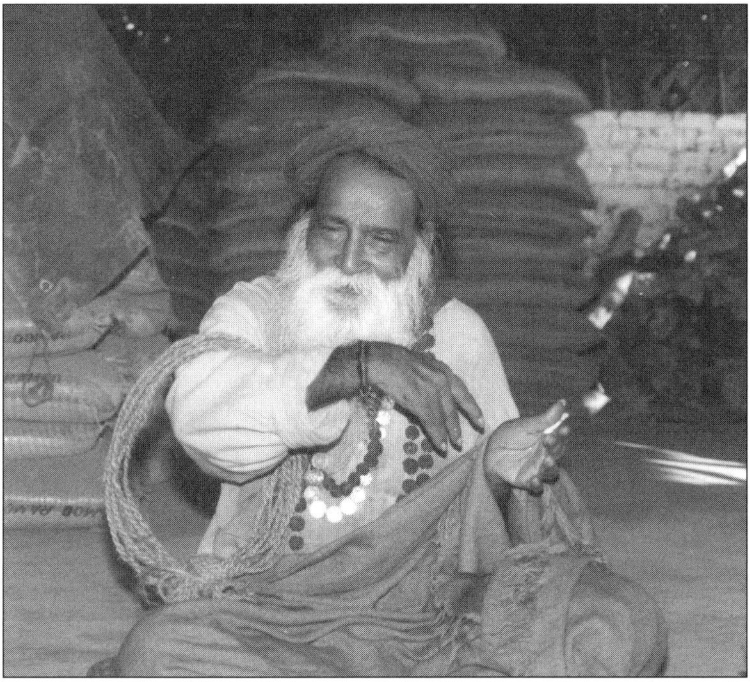

Yogi Ramsuratkumar sits on the ground near the construction site with the rope around his right arm—the same rope used to measure the property for the first time.

In the same way, we can make a covenant with ourselves that no significant obstacle will come between us and our temple building project. In times of conflict and doubt we can remember the teaching that we are essentially *already aligned with the Highest*. We are, on one level, already a temple of God and remembering that will make us ready to manifest our intention in all that we do.

Faith and resolve is at the foundation of one's adhikara, one's covenant with oneself and with the Highest. We strengthen and reflect this resolve by adopting a set of principles and establishing a set of practices that help make our lives sane, grounded and integrated with our heart's vision. This set of foundational principles helps us "touch the ground" optimally in a way that communicates our highest intentions. From this foundational mindset and with these behaviors we are establishing ourselves in building a life of practice and in a profound desire to construct a temple of the body.

Questions to Consider and Write About

1. What does adhikara mean to you?
2. How might you increase your preparedness for your spiritual studies and practice?
3. In what ways is your resolve for building a temple of the body strong?
4. In what ways is your resolve for building a temple of the body weak?
5. In what ways have you experienced the Highest meeting your efforts?
6. What foundational and preliminary actions can you take in your process that will reflect your desire to build a temple of the body?

nine

The Yamas and the Niyamas

Non-violence, truth, abstention from stealing, continence, and absence of greed for possessions beyond one's need are the five pillars of yama.

Yamas are the great, mighty, universal vows, unconditioned by place, time and class.

Cleanliness, contentment, spiritual zeal, self-study and surrender to the Supreme Self or God are the niyamas.

—Yoga Sutras of Patanjali, v. 2:30-2:32

At the foundational level of almost every yoga school are the *yamas* and the *niyamas*, the ethical and moral precepts. In the eight-limbed path of Patanjali's Ashtanga Yoga, they are considered the first two limbs of the path. We see their presence historically as well in streams of Buddhism and Jainism.(1)

The yamas are the moral and ethical precepts which provide the foundation of our practice, and are the bedrock upon which the temple of the body is built. They help guide our efforts by establishing guidelines and principles for conducting ourselves with integrity and maturity.

The yamas are the "don'ts" of yoga, primarily in regards to our relationship with others: Don't harm, don't lie, don't steal, don't misuse your sexual energy and don't hoard. As guidelines they "must be applied on a relative basis to each unique circumstance and context in which the yogi is involved."[2] The niyamas are the yogi's ethical and moral observances primarily in regards to our relationship with ourselves. These are the "do's" of yoga: Be clean, be content, work hard, study the self and offer everything to the Supreme. Generally speaking, the yamas refer more to how one conducts him- or herself in the outer world, within society, and the niyamas refer more to how one conducts him- or herself internally.[3]

The Structure

This chapter begins with a general overview of what these injunctions mean to me. Then, it presents a list of the principles of yama and niyama as outlined by John Friend in the *Anusara Yoga Teacher Training Manual*, in the section called "Classical Ethical Guidelines." It may also be helpful to compare these translations with other commentators for a well-rounded view. Each principle is followed by a few questions that you can use to explore, in a deeper way, what these tenets mean to you and how you might bring them to life to create a stable foundation for your temple construction project. I encourage you to go slowly and work your way through these questions over a period of time. It can also be helpful to review them whenever you feel a bit off balance in your life of practice. Often, when we are feeling out of sorts it is because we have lost some part of our foundation. If we are willing to attend to it, as these questions propose, then foundational sanity, clarity, and stability can be reestablished quite quickly

The questions that follow each brief description of the yamas or niyamas are not intended as accusations or indictments. Instead, they are invitations to explore your personal strengths and weaknesses relative to these qualities and guidelines and to move deeper into the process of self-love that is the deepest yoga.

Foundations and Outcomes

Every one of us acts violently at times—toward ourselves and others—in violation of the yama of *ahimsa* or non-harming. Many of us find it difficult to tell the truth (the yama of truthfulness is known as *satya*)—even if to ourselves, about our anger, our indulgences and our judgments. Most of us are at least occasionally tempted to take what is not ours (as opposed to the yama of *asteya*, non-stealing), even if it is taking just a little bit of credit for something we didn't do. Many times, *brahmacharya* (having God-like ethical conduct) is compromised when the temptation to flirt or to misuse our sexual energy slips into our behavior, especially when we are not paying close attention to our conduct. Rarely have I met someone in our culture who didn't in some way participate in grasping for material objects and using more than they needed, as opposed to the practice of *santosha* (contentment) and *aparigraha* (non-hoarding).

While many people, myself included, often approach these yamas and niyamas as foundational prerequisites of the Path, I see them, in actuality, as foundations *and* outcomes. My own experiences of ahimsa, for instance, illustrate this point.

I came to yoga with a long history of violent behavior toward myself. For many years my relationship with my body was full of harm. I was critical of myself, my body, my personality . . . just about every aspect of who I was and every aspect of my life. From this primary mood of harm, of *himsa*, I acted out violently and self-destructively. I overate. I underate. I over-exercised. I under-exercised. I binged. I purged. I drank too much. I did drugs. I was promiscuous.

While some of the extremes of this cycle had settled down by the time I came to yoga, I still struggled with deep feelings of self-criticism and self-judgment. I was, in truth, quite violent toward myself. (Many of the details of this process are outlined in my first book, *Yoga From the Inside Out*.) Yoga began to plant new seeds of non-harming within me. And by watering those seeds of ahimsa I felt a kind of love for myself grow up in the midst of the self-hatred.

This self-love has since grown to be bigger than the self-hatred. The practice of yoga yielded the experience of self-love that has then made it easier to practice and experience non-violence. Had I been required to be established in ahimsa *before* practicing yoga, there would have been little hope for me of ever glimpsing such peace for myself, or even for practicing yoga. I needed the practice of yoga itself to deliver me, at least in part, to the ability to practice ahimsa. The interplay of yoga practice and the appreciation and expression of ethical principles is a self-perpetuating or reinforcing cycle. As this cycle continues, we find ourselves closer to our true self—where, in our intrinsic goodness, we are already aligned with such high ideals.

I noticed a similar interactive effect in the case of becoming a vegetarian. Practicing yoga for so long, my heart had begun to open, and I began to feel a new connection to animals. I began to feel that killing them for food was harming them, so I cut down on my consumption of meat. Interestingly, the more I refrained from eating meat, the more connected I felt to animals. The more connected I felt to animals, the less I wanted to eat meat. The less I ate meat, the more I recognized my connection to animals . . . and so on. The practice of ahimsa in this domain wasn't imposed from an external rule of "do not harm the animals," but from the recognition of my connection to them brought about through yogic practice.

From this direct experience of connection, being a vegetarian just felt more right for me than eating meat. I believe that every lasting change in behavior and outlook that I have integrated into my life has followed a similar trajectory and process of recognition.

The process of refining oneself relative to foundational principles is ongoing. One of my favorite concepts that Lee Lozowick teaches is that "There is no top end" to practice. We are always invited to refine our practice and the ways we apply *dharmic* principles to our lives.

The Yamas

The yamas (behavior restraints) are ethical guidelines for the yogi pertaining to her relationship with others in society, the outer environment, or nature. All the yamas apply to actions, words and thoughts.

Ahimsa (Non-harming): Loving kindness to others, not blocking or obstructing the flow of nature, compassion, mercy, gentleness.

1. What does ahimsa mean?
2. What does ahimsa mean to you?
3. In what ways do you act or think violently toward yourself or others?
4. What area of your life would benefit from the consistent practice of ahimsa? How?
5. How might you practice ahimsa in this area?

Satya (Truthfulness): Being genuine and authentic to our inner nature, having integrity, honesty, being honorable, not lying, not concealing the truth, not downplaying or exaggerating.

1. What does satya mean?
2. What does satya mean to you?
3. In what ways do you avoid telling the truth? In what circumstances are you most likely to lie?
4. What area of your life would benefit from the consistent application of satya? How?
5. How might you practice satya in this area?

Asteya (Non-stealing): Not taking what is not yours—money, goods or credit. Not robbing people of their own experience and freedom. Non-desire for another's possessions, qualities or status.

1. What does asteya mean?
2. What does asteya mean to you?
3. In what ways do you violate the spirit of asteya? In what circumstances are you most likely to "steal"?
4. What area of your life would benefit from the consistent application of asteya? How?
5. How might you practice asteya in this area?

Brahmacharya (Walking or having ethical conduct like God): Relating to another with unconditional love and integrity, without selfishness or manipulation. Practicing sexual moderation, restraining from sexual misconduct, and avoiding lustful behavior. Celibacy/chastity.

1. What does brahmacharya mean?
2. What does brahmacharya mean to you?
3. In what ways do you violate the spirit of brahmacharya? In what circumstances are you most likely to misuse your sexual or creative energy? Your power?

4. What area of your life would benefit from the consistent application of brahmacharya? How?
5. How might you practice brahmacharya in this area?

The Niyamas

The niyamas (internal restraints) are ethical guidelines for the yogi pertaining to her daily activities; observances of one's own physical appearance, actions, words and thoughts.

Sauca (purity): Cleanliness, orderliness, precision, clarity, balance. Internal and external purification.

1. What does sauca mean?
2. What does sauca mean to you?
3. In what ways do you violate the spirit of sauca?
4. What area of your life would benefit from the consistent application of sauca? How?
5. How might you practice sauca in this area?

Santosha (Contentment): Equanimity, peace, tranquility, acceptance of the way things are.

1. What does santosha mean?
2. What does santosha mean to you?
3. In what ways do you violate the spirit of santosha? In what circumstances are you most likely to feel a lack of contentment?
4. What area of your life would benefit from the consistent application of santosha? How?
5. How might you practice santosha in this area?

Tapas (Heat): Burning desire for reunion with grace expressed though self-discipline, purification, willpower, austerity and patience.

1. What does tapas mean?
2. What does tapas mean to you?
3. In what ways do you lack the necessary tapas or fire in your sadhana?
4. In what ways are you frustrated with the results you have, but fail to apply yourself dynamically to your practice?
5. What area of your life would benefit from more tapas? How?
6. How might you practice tapas in this area?

Svadhyaya (Study of the Self): Self inquiry, mindfulness, self-study, study of the scriptures, chanting and recitation of the scriptures. Searching for the unknown (Divinity) in the known (physical world) and how it relates to you, your true self.

1. What does svadhyaya mean?
2. What does svadhyaya mean to you?
3. In what areas of your life is your practice of svadhyaya weak? In what areas or circumstances is it difficult to study yourself? In what areas are you acting the most mechanically?
4. What area of your life would benefit from more applied svadhyayas? How?
5. How might you practice svadhyaya in this area?

Ishvara Pranidhana (Devotional offering to grace): Surrender to God, open-heartedness, love, "Not my will, but Thy will be done," willingness to serve the Lord.

1. What does ishvara pranidhana mean?
2. What does ishvara pranidhana mean to you?
3. In what circumstances in your life is your practice of ishvara pranidhana weak? In what areas or circumstances is it difficult to make devotional offerings to God?
4. How does ishvara pranidhana relate to control issues?
5. What area of your life would benefit from more applied ishvara pranidhana? How?
6. How might you practice ishvara pranidhana in this area?

ten

The Conditions

The recommended foundation level conditions include both general guidelines for right living and particular forms of discipline we engage daily. All of these are sacred to us, not because we carry a righteous or falsely "holy" attitude about them, but because they are Names of God. When we practice, we speak God's Name. Thus our practices are not simply a form of personal enrichment, but a blessing that enriches the lives of every being on the planet on a daily basis.

—Hohm Sahaj Mandir Study Manual

Regardless of which lineage or tradition you follow, or what yoga you engage, you will find a set of foundational guidelines that cultivate and prepare you; that help create and build your adhikara (preparedness). In the spiritual school of which I am a part, the foundational practices and lifestyle choices are called the "Conditions." If we choose to engage them, these Conditions help us create a firm foundation for our lives as spiritual practitioners. Just by examining ourselves in relationship to these guidelines we gain great insight into who we are, how we live and how we practice. The Conditions are: study, meditation, diet, exercise, right sexuality and right livelihood. As one might expect, many of the yamas and niyamas are reflected in these core practices. Practitioners from traditions as varied as Christianity, Judaism and Buddhism will recognize tenets common to their faiths as well.

The *Hohm Sahaj Mandir Study Manual* says it this way:

> When one looks at most any spiritual tradition one will find as bedrock to that tradition some form of practice. For instance, in the Zen Buddhism community the basic practice is *zazen*, to sit daily in meditation. In the Muslim and Sufi Traditions the daily periodic ritual of prayer keeps one connected to the tradition and to Allah. In the Christian monastic tradition the Divine Office, a series of psalms, is chanted at assigned hours throughout the day. In Fourth Way schools (those esoteric schools which follow in the footsteps of the great Russian mystic G.I. Gurdjieff) the practice of self-observation is of paramount importance to one seriously engaging that system of work on self. *Kirtan* (devotional chanting of the Name of God) is a mainstay of the Hindu tradition. Eastern Bauls have a practice of devotional singing, dancing and begging. It would be hard to distinguish one as a Baul if they did not beg as this is an underlying foundation principle of their spiritual life. The great South Indian saint Ramana Maharshi instructed his devotees in a form of enquiry centered around the question, "Who am I?" And on it goes.[(1)]

An examination of each of these basic Conditions as they are practiced within the Western Baul tradition will comprise the bulk of this chapter. Perhaps they will encourage you to contemplate and review the foundations upon which you hope to erect your great temple, and upon which you intend to build a life of practice.

Study

> *The more you study about God and the laws of this Work, clarifying your own confusions, and confirming your own experience through Traditions, the more likely it will be that you are laying the foundation for living a life perfectly aligned with the Will of God.*
>
> —Lee Lozowick

While yoga is essentially an experiential subject, in which the practitioner is not concerned with understanding the truth as much as experiencing the truth, study is an important foundational practice. As much as we may have high aspirations and deep longings to align ourselves and our lives with the flow of the Highest, to build of ourselves a temple of the body, we need to know the how of the process. Study helps us to understand the process in which we are involved, gives us time-honored maps and signposts along the way, and helps us see our efforts in relationship to a larger body of practice and tradition. Study is one of the means by which we educate ourselves to participate skillfully in a life of practice, and one way we can make use of the wisdom that has been accumulated by people who have walked the path before us.

Yoga is a very intimate experience for many people. Because of the nature of the endeavor and the deep places it opens within many of us, the process feels extremely personal. Many times we get so involved in our own process that we lose the perspective that our immediate challenges and victories are part of a larger trajectory of growth and transformation. We do not see that, as unique as our challenges seem to us, they are common, in most ways, to the challenges that every sincere practitioner has faced. By studying the different yoga traditions, as well as the lives and works of great practitioners, we can see a bigger picture of sadhana. This bigger vision can help us maintain the proper perspective along the way, seeing that the small ups and downs are simply part of the journey.

Lee Lozowick hit the point this way:

> When one is rightly educated, one finds it easier to accept one's natural state of being. When one is not rightly educated, and that one experiences his or her natural state of being, he or she usually freaks out, terrified of the intensity and vastness of their perceptions.
>
> When one is educated properly it is more likely that one can deal with experience as it arises very simply and spontaneously, with joy. When one is not educated properly, one typically gets depressed or elated when different experiences arise. Either way, high or low, it doesn't matter for either response is a reaction, rather than a natural acceptance of "what is."[(2)]

Another boon of study is that it requires us, as students, to be active participants in our education, which is highly empowering. Instead of being passive recipients of knowledge, we are actively engaging the Path. As important as I believe teachers are, they are limited in what they can teach us if we are not doing our fair share of the work as students.

Early in my yoga studies, I told my yoga instructor that I was having trouble learning the Sanskrit names for the postures. I asked her if she had any suggestions for how to learn them. She looked me squarely in the eye, paused, and replied, "When you care enough, you will learn them." I remember being taken aback. I had expected her to say, "Make flash cards" or "Buy this book" or even "I will help you." But she said, in effect, "Study." I have always been grateful for her response because it put the responsibility for learning on me, where it belonged.

Whether it is the study of the names of the *asanas*, the principles of sequencing poses, or the finer points of yoga philosophy, there is a wealth of information available to expand our knowledge and to deepen our practice of study. Every major yoga school has a required reading list and an even longer list of recommended reading, which can launch one quite well into the fascinating world of study.

In developing a practice of study it can be enormously helpful to set aside a formal period of time. Instead of just lying on the couch and reading a yoga book, I suggest committing yourself to a set period of time, sitting at your desk or in front of your altar, and bringing an intentional quality to your study. Take notes. Do some reflective writing based on what you are reading. If study is a new area of practice for you, start with a formal period of fifteen minutes a few times a week; then increase the time and frequency as you feel ready.

Meditation

Don't believe everything you think.
—Bumper Sticker

I practice an open form of meditation that Lee Lozowick taught me and that is practiced on his ashrams. There are, however, many methods of meditation and many ways to practice its principles. There is focus-type meditation, mantra-based meditation, breath-based meditation as well as a myriad of witness-based techniques that can be employed. For formal meditation instruction, in terms of these various ways and means, I suggest seeking help from an experienced teacher who is trained by an authoritative source and who is designated by his or her teacher as one who is competent to guide others in the practice of meditation.

One thing that meditation can teach us is to observe what Lee Lozowick calls the "endless machinations of the mind." Each one of us has a constant stream of thoughts running through our minds at any given time. Many of these thoughts we are aware of, many of them we are not. Meditation, as I practice it, is not so much the attempt to stop these thoughts as it is an opportunity to see them for what they are. In seeing thoughts for what they are, as endless machinations of the mind, a distance from one's thoughts is established. This distance gives us the space necessary to stop believing everything we think.

Through meditation, we can see that we have different aspects of personality within ourselves, each with its own thoughts. We can learn that even though we think something and it feels *real* to us, the thought may not actually be an accurate representation of our truest reality. Getting to know ourselves in this way is significantly helpful because, then, when these different personality aspects surface in our relationships and in our other endeavors, we are no longer dealing with a stranger but with someone we know pretty well. We can actually learn the ways that our thoughts and feelings tend to distort the reality of our most essential self. This learning will prepare us to avoid making unconscious assumptions about life, one another, or situations in which we find ourselves.

For instance, there might be an aspect of ourselves that always feels victimized and whose tendency is to assign blame rather than take responsibility. If we are not familiar with this aspect of ourselves, we will not recognize her when she is in charge. When she is in control, life seems very personal, unfair, and out to get us. From this position, people's motives will be suspect and our decision-making process, our relationships and our feelings about life in general will be founded on a distorted version of what is actually going on. We will be living not in "life as it is" but in an unconscious psychological projection of how life is.

Weeding through these psychological projections and creating the ability to observe what we are thinking develops within us the power of discernment and discrimination. In order to build a temple of the body we must become aware of our thoughts so that we can have the power of choice in relationship to them. For example, if we eat something every time we think about food, then we are reacting to our thoughts as if they are directives for action, not simply thoughts about food. If every time we are just a little too hot we have to turn on the air conditioning, we are reacting as though the thoughts indicating discomfort contained an imperative to action.

In those moments, our meditation practice can come to life so that we can *choose* our actions rather than simply reacting habitually from these unconscious imperatives. If we have spent time in meditation seeing our thoughts as simply thoughts, and getting to know our typical reactions to discomfort, psychological fear and/or physical cravings, we are better prepared to choose a response to our life circumstances rather than succumb to unconscious reaction. This moment of choice is the moment in which we become practitioners. In these moments of conscious choice we are building a temple of the body rather than unconsciously strengthening our body of habits. These are moments where the space and clarity of what we learn in meditation can teach us a lot.

These insights and options are only part of the great opportunity of meditation. For, after years of seeing the endless machinations of the mind for what they are, the practice of meditation begins to point us toward *what we are*. We glimpse the deeper layers of the self and become more established in our inner life.

Seven Simple Guidelines for Meditation

As a foundational practice, meditation is most effective when at least a few principles are followed.

1. Regardless of the meditation technique that you practice, practice one technique consistently. Don't jump around trying out new approaches from one day to the next. This consistency will give you a chance to understand what any one technique has to offer.
2. If at all possible, establish a regular time to practice so that meditation becomes a regular part of your day. This will also condition your body/mind in a way that predisposes you toward meditation like a positive habit.
3. Set a timer to determine the length of your meditation practice, and stay for the duration. Learn to simply observe the wanting to get up as a thought that requires no action. If you merely meditate until you feel like you are "done," then you miss a valuable opportunity to observe yourself.
4. The ten minutes that you practice is better than the sixty minutes that you do not practice. So if you need to start small, or if some days you have less time, simply do what you can. Keeping a consistency in this area will prove beneficial.

5. Sit up straight, but do not obsess about your posture. Occasionally checking in as you sit is sufficient.
6. Breathe normally, through your nose, if possible.
7. Enjoy yourself. As my teacher Lee Lozowick says, "You know, meditation should be fun. It shouldn't be this heavy thing, like 'everyday I've got to meditate, or else I'm doomed.' It should be light and joyful, interesting, fascinating and productive."(3)

Diet

Success comes to a person of faith and self-confidence, but there is not success for others. Hence, practice hard. The first sign of success is confidence that one's efforts will bear fruit. The second is being firm in that faith; the third is worship of the guru; the fourth is equanimity; the fifth is control over the senses; the sixth is moderate eating; there is no seventh.

—Georg Feuerstein

We are a culture absolutely obsessed with diet. As much as we are hoping some diet or food plan will be the answer, we are often rebellious, opinionated and resistant to making changes in our longstanding beliefs, opinions and habits around food. People in the affluent Western world are swinging from extremes of unhealthy thinness and eating disorders to obesity, which has hit epidemic proportions in the U.S. Clearly, food is an area in which many of us are struggling to find balance.

I believe that no one system of diet will work for everyone. In fact, the reasons that we diet are quite varied. Some of us are overweight, some are underweight. Some people are struggling with anxiety, others with depression. Some of us have health concerns that call for specialized food plans. Some live alone and have a simple quiet life; others live in the midst of great stress and interact with a lot of different people. People in colder climates will need different foods in the middle of the winter than those who live in the tropics. These variables are endless.

While I will not offer a diet plan, or make recommendations about specific foods in this book, I will assert that food—and more specifically one's relationship to food—is a seriously important area to review. After I wrote *Yoga From the Inside Out* I got many phone calls and letters from people who had struggled with eating disorders and body image issues in much the same way as I had. By phone, email or in personal conversations we would talk about the book, sharing our similar and different stories and experiences. After a period of sharing, quite often the reader would say something to me like, "Yes, I know that self-love is important, but *what should I eat*?"

The questions would always jar me a bit. I would think, "I don't know what you should eat!" I wrote my first book to explain to myself and others that the problem (food, body image, eating disorders, self-hatred, etc.) was a spiritual dilemma and that no food plan or number on the scale or dress size was ever going to fix a problem that was essentially spiritual. In my opinion, the answer—the only lasting peace—will come from realizing that we are asking questions such as "How can I get thinner?" and "What should I eat?" when we should be asking questions like "What is my purpose?", "How can I serve?" and "Does my life glorify God and honor the essential goodness that is at the heart of everything?"

Having said that, I do know from direct experience that when my relationship with food is tipped to an extreme, it is difficult for me to contemplate higher concerns like service and devotion. And because the question of what to eat so often accompanied a person's deep personal sharing about his or her own struggles, I know food is a big and important topic to address. I also know from experience that the content of my diet does matter. What I choose to eat and choose not to eat can have a dramatic effect on my physical health, my weight and my general vitality as well as my mental and emotional outlook. In many ways, the body is a chemical machine. Different foods affect the chemistry of the machine and its balance differently. And, it will serve each one of us to learn about that balance directly.

Ayurveda . . . or Not

I have found a lot of help from the principles of Ayurveda and by working directly with an Ayurvedic physician to determine a diet appropriate to my personal health needs and temperament. Ayurveda has a long history and tradition and is considered yoga's sister science. Its efficacy has stood the test of time; it is not a fad diet that will be disproven next year when some new research comes out.

Central to the Ayurveda regime is the idea of *doshas* or personal types. Diets, exercise strategies and lifestyle practices are recommended relative to an individual's type and specific situation. This approach explains a lot about why some people have success on food plans that prove disastrous to others.

As much as I love the Ayurvedic approach to diet and health, Ayurveda is not by any means a formal recommendation or a requirement for success in stabilizing a foundational relationship to food. For many, even the basic practices of Ayurveda would be difficult to implement. The appropriate diet for anyone will depend on where they are starting from relative to food, diet, physical health, and what their specific goals are. For instance, if your diet is largely meat-based, a dramatic shift to a vegetarian diet may prove too drastic. If your current diet is made up of fast food, meals in restaurants and convenience-oriented menus then the likelihood of being successful on a plan that consists of whole-foods cooked at home would be slim. The change required would quite likely feel too extreme and might prove to be a set-up for future rebellion or backsliding. Additionally, certain strict plans can work against someone with an eating disorder because they can tend to reinforce the neurotic rule-based relationship one may already have with food. Additionally, in emphasizing diet, we run the risk of looking to a diet to solve problems of the mind and heart, when dietary practices are a tool and a practice, not a solution to anything.

A Different Relationship to Food

Early in my recovery with bulimia I worked with a nutritionist who was renowned for natural healing through whole foods, and for recommending pure diets to his patients. He began our consultation by asking me about my history with food. As I shared with him some of my story he put down his pad and listened attentively. At the end he told me, "You get a very special plan. For you, your aim is to eat from all the food groups in moderation with no 'outlawed' food." He explained to me that my focus should be just on feeling reasonably normal about eating and that to impose a lot of do's and don'ts would be counterproductive since I felt so weird and "special" already. We worked together on portion control, on what appropriate amounts of various foods were. He suggested that I stay away from foods laden with artificial sweeteners and chemicals as they would not be helpful in establishing a physical balance. He recommended that I eat real foods, not diet foods, and that I should move from thinking I could eat more of something simply because it was labeled "low-calorie" or "light."

That interview stayed with me for a long time, and for many years I worked with his advice to expand my relationship with food to be more inclusive and less restrictive. From that vantage point I began to see that certain foods were easier than others to be moderate with, and that it would be in my best interest to not eat certain foods that I couldn't help but binge on. This is an entirely different context than seeing food as good or bad.

If we hope to make a temple of the body then we must recognize that the food we put into our body is of the utmost importance and any movement we can make toward establishing a healthy eating regime will be beneficial to our task.

Four Types of Hunger

Regardless of the content of one's diet, it is crucial to get a handle on portion amounts and to train oneself to understand and to respond appropriately to what I call the four types of hunger: physical hunger, mouth hunger, emotional hunger and spiritual hunger.

Physical hunger is the hunger the body feels when it needs food or fuel. Just as a car needs gas to run, so too the body needs fuel in the form of food. In this domain it makes prefect sense to eat food that is wholesome, free from chemicals and as close to its natural state as possible.

Mouth hunger is simply the pleasure we feel in our mouths, through our taste buds, that makes us want to keep eating even when our physical hunger is satisfied. It is also what helps us to experience joy in eating and to *love what we eat* as well as to *eat what we love*. Both sides of the coin are important, and no success will come with diet unless the food we eat is largely satisfying and enjoyable. In fact, enjoyment is seen as an important aspect of Ayurveda. According to this approach, the mood with which we eat is as vital, if not more so, as what we eat.

Emotional hunger drives us to eat rather than feel. Sometimes it is mouth hunger that keeps us eating. We take a second helping because it tastes so good, not because we are physically hungry. But many times we eat more than our bodies require because there is some kind of emotional discomfort that arises when we are no longer in the act of eating. Perhaps we feel awkward sitting at the table, finished with our meal, while other people continue to eat. That feeling of awkwardness goes away if we keep eating, so we continue eating instead of staying with our discomfort. Maybe we eat when we are in our house alone instead of remaining present to our feelings of loneliness. Maybe we simply cannot endure the feeling of desire, the feeling of wanting some tasty food, without acting out on the urge. The variations to this theme are endless, but the point is that we can learn to recognize and respond to emotional signals to eat as distinct from physical hunger signals. Emotional hunger cannot be fed with physical food. It must be fed by honestly acknowledging our emotions and by working with them and/or expressing them in healthy ways.

Spiritual hunger is the hunger we feel for a life of dignity, joy and true purpose. Spiritual hunger is the hunger to serve something greater than ourselves, the hunger to realize our true self, and the hunger for our small concerns to be subsumed by a larger vision. Spiritual hunger is the hunger for our highest ideals to be manifested in our lives. We might be hungry to know our purpose and place in the world, or perhaps we feel this hunger as burning zeal for enlightenment. Spiritual hunger leads us to prayer, to acts of devotion, to moving beyond our comfort zone in order to satisfy this profound craving. Like emotional hunger, spiritual hunger cannot be satisfied with a second helping, or a bowl (or even a gallon) of premium ice cream; and even the best chef in the world cannot make a meal rich enough to fill us up in this way. We must feed this hunger with what will be ultimately satisfying.

Impression Food

In Part I, Chapter 5, we discussed the different sheaths of the body, acknowledging that we are multilayered beings. With this understanding, we can expand our idea of food and diet to include a multidimensional aspect as well. Just as we take in food we also take in impressions from the world. And just as healthy food nourishes the body and unhealthy food contributes to the body's breakdown, the diet of psychic impressions that we consume nourishes our inner life or contributes to its malfunctioning. Violent movies; sexually demeaning images; sensationalist media programming; negative thoughts about ourselves, our lives and/or one another; all become food for our psychological, psychic and subtle bodies. Learning what is good nutrition in these domains is as important as knowing what one should eat for dinner. Maybe more so.

My Ayurvedic physician once remarked to me that he cannot understand why so many people worry about a cup of coffee a day and pay no attention to what they watch on television, what they read in the paper or what they talk about. We owe it to ourselves to evaluate the diet of impressions that feed our minds and hearts, as well as the diet we feed our physical body. Finding nourishing food on all levels goes a long way toward building a reliable foundation for a life of practice.

Questions to Consider and Write About

1. What is your current relationship with food?

2. What does emotional hunger mean to you?
3. Spiritually, what are you most hungry for?
4. What are some impression foods that will ultimately satisfy your spiritual hunger and what are the ones that help keep your hunger gnawing?

Exercise

> *Lack of activity destroys the good condition of every human being, while movement and methodical physical exercise save it and preserve it.*
>
> —Plato

The body is designed to move. As a foundational practice, daily exercise helps keep our body fit, strong and conditioned, thus aligning the body with its design for movement. Just as many people in our culture have an extreme (i.e., unbalanced) relationship with food, so they also have with exercise. On one end of the spectrum is the tendency toward a fully sedentary lifestyle—we spend more time at computers, in cars and sitting at desks than we do up and about playing sports or even just walking to the store. On the other end of the spectrum is a trend toward over-exercising and wearing the body down through overuse, in the vain attempt to attain an unrealistic physique.

Exercise as a foundational practice is not about fitness or about whipping ourselves into shape. Daily exercise is about aligning ourselves with what the body needs for health in a sane and mature way as an act of loving worship. Caring for the body—which is an expression of the Divine as well as the vehicle through which we will practice, worship and serve—is so much more than a fitness plan.

About this subject Lee Lozowick writes:

> Our physical body is designed to function under a certain level of stress. This healthy stress, which has both qualitative and quantitative elements, is generally either ignored or exceeded in our contemporary culture. Regular physical exercise is a very natural way to balance the body's stress level, and to enhance the flow of vital energy, but too much physical exercise, or the wrong type can actually be quite destructive. When the body is balanced and vitalized, the emotions and mind tend to come into balance as well, creating an optimum resonance with "Already Present Enlightenment" in a mood of alertness and dynamism.
>
> Our condition of exercise is designed to maintain a body that communicates the essence of Elegance . . . This includes tone of the body, brightness of the body, which is its process of conductive life energy (or *shakti* or *chi* in other words) and posture. This all requires a body that is strong and has stamina and yet is supple, vibrant and alive. Such a body is in a state of relaxed sensitivity, optimally available and alert to the environment and Divine Influence.(4)

For me, and I assume for many reading this book, yoga asana practice is one of my primary forms of exercise. Yoga is unparalleled in its ability to increase physical strength and suppleness as well as metal focus, clarity and concentration. We cultivate our attention, we learn to observe ourselves and we develop the ability to manage our minds and emotions, all while strengthening, stretching and celebrating the body.

Asana practice trains our attention on many levels: We learn to pay attention to the body and breath as we attend to the details of our alignment and to the forms of the postures themselves. In this process, our mind is getting trained to focus and our ability to concentrate improves. We learn, just as we do in meditation, to witness strong sensations without reacting to or immediately acting on our feelings. By increasing our sensitivity, paying attention and by quieting ourselves in practice we learn to objectively observe what is happening in our emotional life. Sometimes old feelings surface as the body releases stored tensions; sometimes the time out from normal life provides enough space for our emotions to surface in an uncompensated and unrationalized state. Bringing the body into alignment can also bring our emotions into a state of alignment and integrity. The more skilled we become as practitioners who can recognize the truth and joy of who we essentially are, the more we can work with our emotions by keeping them in the context of a larger picture of being.

Just as the body, the mind and the emotions become a focus of our attention, so too does the life of the spirit. As we noted in Part I, Chapter 7, "prana follows attention" so the ability to attend skillfully to each of these various domains will help us considerably in our overall effort to build a temple of the body. As we hone our ability to attend skillfully to the various demands and opportunities in asana practice, we are honing our ability to attend to the demands and opportunities that life and our sadhana will undoubtedly present to us.

Instead of looking at yoga (or any other exercise for that matter) simply as a workout or a fitness modality, we can use it to establish ourselves in the foundational context of practice. Yoga, particularly when it uses heart-inspiring themes that help the practitioner to physicalize virtue, provides an excellent way to bring this foundational context to life. In building a temple of the body, the conscious use of metaphor will help us remember our deeper purposes, thus placing our exercise regime in the domain of practice and worship. For instance, spending our practice time consciously focusing on the way our foundation is placed in each asana rather than just going through the motions mechanically can help us embody our ideal of building our temple on solid ground. After an hour or two of such intentional focus, we will be less likely to step off the yoga mat or a treadmill and forget our true, foundational intentions.

A Genuine Regular Practice

In order to use our asana practice as a means to sanctify the body, we must *have* a regular practice. Perhaps those struggling to establish a practice will find inspiration by connecting to a high purpose for their endeavor. Perhaps even longtime practitioners can find deeper levels and renewal from such a potent context of using asana practice to lay a strong foundation in building a temple of the body. I cannot stress enough the importance of personal practice in this process of building a temple. And, in this case, I am making a clear distinction between a genuine personal practice and simply attending yoga classes.

I love yoga classes. I love to teach them. I love to take them. I have found great benefit from attending classes regularly. I also love workshops, intensives and trainings. I particularly love group practices where seasoned practitioners join together to practice. Each of these expressions of yoga has so much to offer the participant. But there are distinct differences between personal practice, group practice, and taking classes, workshops and trainings. The more each of us can be aware of what the differences are, the more we can increase the benefit of these differences and minimize the liability of each format.

After I wrote *Yoga From the Inside Out* I got several letters complaining that "no one talks about this stuff in classes," meaning that, no one talks about how yoga practice is a way of confronting self-hatred and making peace with our body. I wrote the book hoping that people would take the ideals of self-love, self honor and paying attention into their personal practice, integrate these concepts and then hold them as a guiding internal context in classes or other group situations.

That same hope applies to the material presented here. As you begin to incorporate the ideas from this book into practice, please take responsibility for them by bringing them to life in your own practice first. In fact, if this book served no other function but to help you roll out a sticky mat at home three times a week, that would be high praise for its value.

The importance of good instruction and community cannot be overstated. But, there is a sanctuary to be found in personal practice that no class or workshop provides. There is a sense of empowerment that comes when you know that you are reliable in your commitment to practice, in your own personal time of self-exploration and experimentation; something that classes cannot offer. In a personal practice, in the intimacy of your own breath as it joins your heart's intention, alone with yourself, you can establish your foundation and begin to build a temple of the body, a life of practice and a sanctuary for your self that is there for you at all time and in all places.

Right Relationship and Sexuality

> *A life of practice . . . when one is in a coupled situation includes a full, rich, lusty and deeply relational and honoring sexual communion, genitally and energetically.*
>
> —Lee Lozowick

The Condition of right relationship and sexuality as a foundational practice invites us to pay attention to the ways that we manage our most primal urges and needs for intimacy, connection and sexual union.

While classical yoga traditions often recommended celibacy and a life of renunciation (*brahmacharya*), the tantric practitioners regarded sex as a part of embodied life not separate from the Supreme Consciousness, and therefore another way through which to honor, celebrate, and affirm the immanence of the Divine. Anyone who researches tantra will soon come across references to sexual rituals and practices that can seem quite startling. Some texts even reference having sex with corpses! While sexual rites are certainly a part of some tantric schools and sects, the modern associations and interpretations are misleading and, for the most part, represent a distorted misunderstanding of the context, intention and principles behind these esoteric practices. Sexuality as part of spiritual life is not a free for all of indulgence or a set of techniques to achieve multiple orgasms. Sexuality within a life of practice is a means by which we affirm the presence of the Highest in and through the body and in relationship to another person who shares this same context.

As with its behaviors regarding food and exercise, our contemporary culture is full of unhealthy extremes in the domain of sex and relationship. Many people are so bound up they cannot enjoy this natural expression of life. Others act out in such distorted ways that any link to the sacred is out of the question. Bringing ourselves into a healthy balance is where we should focus our attention as modern practitioners of tantra, not on rituals dating back to the tenth century and earlier, that often had to do with esoteric ideas of alchemy.

Examining ourselves and practicing in the domain of relationship and sexuality is first and foremost a question of energy management. Sexual energy is potent energy and, as practitioners dedicated to bringing the Divine to life through the body, the way we manage ourselves relative to this potent transformational force deserves our attention. The more potent an energy is, the greater the opportunity it provides for our transformation and revelation, but also the more temptation it provides into deeper levels of cloaking. In the Western Baul tradition, Lee Lozowick has always recommended monogamous, committed relationships as foundational expressions of this Condition, saying, "The basic Condition of sexuality in our Community centers around energy management. Monogamy (having one partner) is recommended over 'playing the field,' and any sexual involvement should be based on a real sense of commitment to communion in relationship, not simply on animal drives."[(5)]

Each of us will need to find an expression of sexuality that best honors our true purpose of building a temple of the body and a life of practice. And just as different diets and asana are appropriate for different types of people, sexual relationships may vary a bit from person to person relative to age, sexual orientation and personality. If we look honestly at right relationship and right sexuality in the light of energy management, we can see that time spent flirting, game playing, seducing others, and playing the field, all of which are common in our culture, and may be fun for many, are expenditures of energy that may not serve us in deepening our life of practice. Simply stated, energy that is wrapped up solely in the pursuit of sex and its accompanying gratifications is energy not available for a life of worship.

While this formula sounds simple, I know it is not necessarily easy to get a handle on optimal energy management. Even questioning ourselves in this domain, much less making any real change that might be needed, can be difficult because we are bombarded constantly and throughout our entire lives with overt and often times inappropriate sexual images and messages. We are not trained to see our attitudes and/or behaviors clearly in this domain, nor to hold an optimal context. Furthermore, different religions and cultures have unique views regarding sexuality. Careful questioning and rigorous self-honesty will be our best assets in establishing a solid foundation in right sexuality and relationship. Staying connected to our intention of putting the Highest first and increasing our sensitivity helps to assist this objective process of self inquiry and exploration.

If you find yourself frequently obsessing, worrying, acting out and/or making choices about sex or relationship that result in painful outcomes, this area is worthy of your attention. If you are in a monogamous relationship but you find little enjoyment in sex, also consider this domain as worthy of your attention. All of us can profit from reviewing how we are aligned with chosen values, rather than with society's norms.

Questions to Consider and Write About

1. What is your relationship to sex?
2. How would you like that relationship to be?
3. In what ways does your sexuality feel aligned with your desire to build a temple of your body? In what ways does is seem misaligned?

Right Livelihood

Work is love made visible.

—Kahlil Gibran

I consider it a great fortune to be earning my living by teaching yoga. I love the subject matter, the challenge of working with different types of people and the opportunity to grow and learn as a student and a teacher. Teaching yoga gives me the opportunity to immerse myself in the teachings of the tradition of which I am a part, and to be in a constant consideration of yogic principles and philosophies. However, one of my favorite things about yoga is that people from all walks of life practice it. People of all professions join together in this practice and become unified through the practice and principles of this great art and science.

Examining our issues of right livelihood relative to building a temple of the body is simply to examine whether how we earn a living is aligned, in a general way, with our chosen values and ethics. If we find ourselves involved in a career or job that is at odds with our deepest values, chances are that this conflict will work against our efforts of building a life of spiritual practice.

It is also important to examine the attitudes we have about our work. Often I talk to people who are not so happy with their work and find it less than inspiring or meaningful. They dream about more meaningful work, often missing the value of the work they are already doing. Even a job that we are not passionate about, but which provides us a good living and a reliable means to care for ourselves and others, can be seen as a valuable foundation upon which to build a life of practice. The practices of looking for the good and putting the Highest first can help us start to appreciate our work in a different way.

Right livelihood does not necessarily mean that we *love* our job, or that it is our bliss, or any such romantic notion. If that happens to be our story . . . well, *great*! But if not, perhaps our job may be the means by which we finance our deeper passions: like giving us the resources to pursue our love of yoga or anything that brings us closer to the highest ideals of our heart.

Money

> Sometimes when the cash-flow was short of what we needed in the next week to buy materials, I would go to Bhagwan and tell Him, "The flow is less than what we need. Can you bless me Bhagwan? This is your Father's work. Can you ask Him to provide the funds?" We always built according to what we had available. The money came just as we needed it. This was always the case.—Mani, *A Man and His Master*, 198

Examining how we spend our money falls under this Condition of right livelihood as well. If we want to build a life of practice but are frittering our money away on entertaining indulgences, we have the opportunity to shore up that part of our foundation. Perhaps we love to go out for a night on the town, every weekend, and yet we have no money to attend the yoga workshops and classes that we say we want to go to. Perhaps we spend so much money on clothes and fancy shoes that we cannot afford to take time off for spiritual renewal or physical rejuvenation. We might find, upon our review, that we are spending much of our time and energy (in the form of money) on an extravagant lifestyle that keeps us on a treadmill of overwork. On the flipside, we might be so afraid of hard work that we do not apply ourselves to our capacity and are chronically in debt, without necessary funds to pursue rewarding endeavors. We may habitually live closer to the bone than necessary.

Again, how much money we make and what we spend it on is not so much the point. Rather, this condition is about the context we bring to our work and our relationship with money so that it moves from an unconscious act into the realm of conscious, skillful participation. If we align our relationship with our money and our work with the highest ideals of the heart, we truly strengthen the foundation of our temple of the body.

Questions to Consider and Write About

1. In what ways does your work support your sadhana?
2. How would you describe your relationship with your work?
3. Can you see the ultimate value of the work you do? For instance, maybe your work is of great value to someone else or to the world in some way.
4. What does your work enable you to enjoy?
5. What are the ways in which your relationship to money is supporting your alignment with your highest ideals? And in what ways is it hindering your alignment?

PART III

SCAFFOLDING: ERECTING AND MAINTAINING WALLS OF SUPPORT

Having considered a foundational mindset and what it takes to build a strong and reliable foundation, we are now ready to examine how the scaffolding for the temple is created and what it does.

Strong supportive walls will uphold us as we build a temple of the body through a life of practice. When we practice asana we create a muscular tone that aids and protects the muscles in the performance of the pose. In the same way, off the mat we create a strong tone by skillfully engaging the muscles of the *dharma*/the teaching, the *guru*/the spiritual authority and the *kula*/the community and by cultivating enthusiastic discipline.

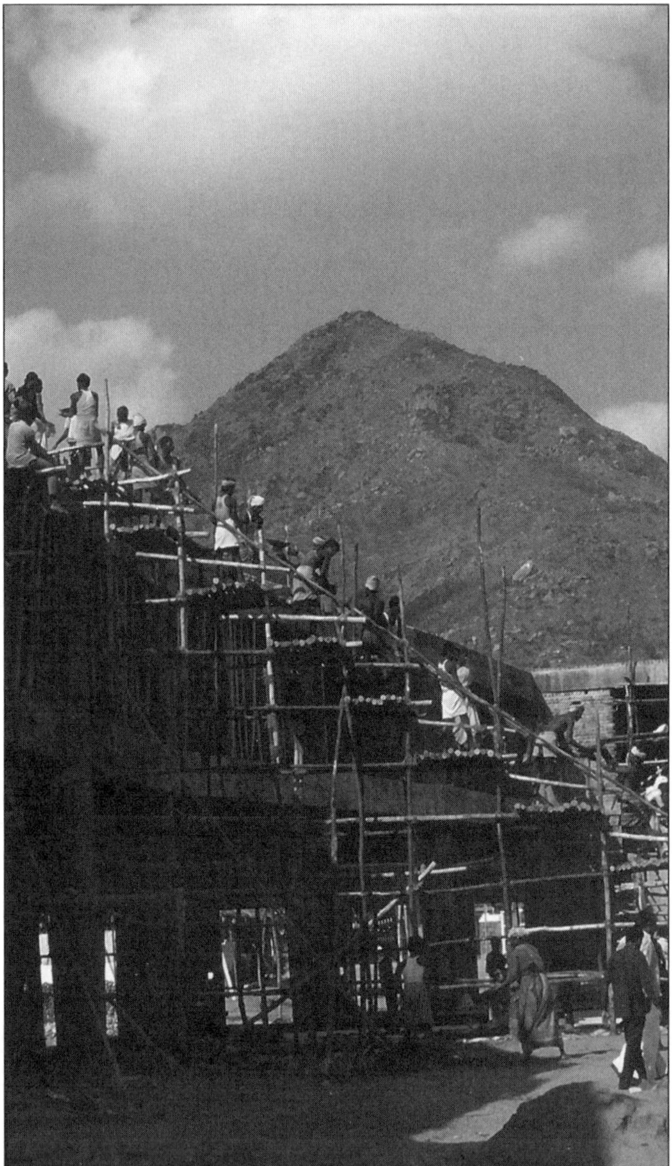

Temple workers climb the intricate scaffolding in the construction of the Temple of Yogi Ramsuratkumar, Tiruvannamalai, India, 1997. Mount Arunachala blesses all.

eleven

The Dharma

By knowing the One, we know everything
—The Vedas

The Sanskrit word *dharma* literally means "that which sustains and upholds" and is therefore part of the supportive scaffolding of the temple of the body and our life of practice. Often translated as "duty" or "virtue," dharma also means "the teachings of the truth" or the "science of religious duty."

In his commentary on the Yoga Sutras of Pantajali, B.K.S. Iyengar writes: "*Dharma* is that which upholds, sustains, and supports one who has fallen or is falling, or is about to fall in the sphere of ethics, physical or mental practices, or spiritual discipline."(1) Defined in this way, we see that the dharma is for all of us. Certainly, each one of us can identify with at least one of these spheres! Who among us has not fallen, is not falling right now, or might not fall in the future? And even if we are perfectly moral in our behavior, perhaps our mental life is out of sync with our righteous behavior. We might actually be doing the right things for the wrong reasons.

Depending on our religious affiliation, upbringing and beliefs, the dharma or the teaching by which we live may seem to vary slightly in content or in mood from that of other people.

In essence, however, dharma is grounded in the principles that *unify* all religions, not in the distinctions and differences among traditions. Building a temple of the body through yoga is not at odds with practicing Christianity, Judaism or Buddhism, for example, because the spirit of the task, the context of the endeavor, is not defined by ideology or creed.

Elsewhere, Iyengar writes:

> Dharma is not about denomination or cult. It is universal...Dharma is about the search for enduring ethical principles, about the cultivation of right behavior in physical, moral, mental, psychological and spiritual dimensions. This behavior must always relate to the growth of the individual with the goal of realizing the Soul. If it does not, if it is culturally limited or warped, then it falls short of the definition of dharma. Sadhana, the practitioner's inward journey, admits of no barriers between individuals, cultures, races, or creeds. So neither can dharma. The discovery of the Universal Soul through the realization of the individual Soul is an experience that, by definition, can leave no frontiers intact. I do not object to the word religion—I am used to it—but some people do. So let us just remember that the earliest Latin root of the word religion—*religare*—means to be aware, and absolute awareness will never perceive difference or conflict. Only partial awareness can do that. Most religious people are therefore only partially religious. That implies that however good their intentions, they still need an even fuller, more inclusive awareness.(2)

Having a good road map for the journey, that is, understanding the dharma and understanding how these larger teachings apply to any specific path in life, can support and uphold us in the midst of the many choices and challenges we face in the process of erecting a temple of the body in a world where the body is often objectified or ignored and even abused and disregarded. For those of us building a temple of the body, understanding these teachings is like getting to see the blueprints of the great architect! Such an overview provides us great insight into the necessity and value of all the building materials for the project.

The Highest

As we have highlighted throughout this book, the principle of putting the Highest first is bedrock. In this chapter, therefore, let's be clear that the fundamental reason why we study dharmic teachings, and why we explore the ways that the Divine functions, is to increase our knowledge of and our skill at putting the Highest first. In this way we optimize our efforts to align with and even merge with the Highest.

Knowledge of the nature of the Highest is a supportive structure for those of us wanting to build a temple of the body. After all, how can we build a temple of the body that is a *dedicated to the Highest*, *made possible by the Highest* and is essentially *an expression of the Highest*, if we are fuzzy or uninformed about what the Highest actually is? The truth is we can't. We need the dharma for this. Dharma is truly that which supports and upholds us because it gives us direction, focus and information about how to proceed optimally in the flow of the Highest.

While each religious tradition has a dharma that elaborates the distinctions of its creed, we will use the language of one that has been useful for me—Kashmir Shaivism—and one that is often applied in hatha yoga instruction. The dharma of Kashmir Shaivism considers the nature of the Highest and the essence of all life and its functions in the light of thirty-six principles of truth, known as *tattvas*. These tattvas are also sometimes referred to as principles of being or principles of nature. At first, this extensive series of dharmic distinctions, with their Sanskrit names, can be a bit daunting, especially for those of us in the West who were raised within a Judeo-Christian cosmology. Nonetheless, I have found this exploration of tattvas to be useful as a road map for the inner journey. To simply read over these ideas may help you to gain insight into your life and your self. A schematic of the tattvas is found in the Appendix, page 195.

The Tattvas

The Supreme, as a unifying, all-pervading consciousness and energy breaks down and expresses itself through thirty-six different *tattvas*, or principles of truth, being and/or nature. The *tattvas* are categorized into various stages of consciousness and manifestations so that we might understand these unifying principles more deeply. The tattvas are quite orderly, and offer us great insight into the nature of the greater cosmos as well as the microcosm of our personal experience.

Central to these teachings is the concept of one divine energy or supreme consciousness that informs everything else, and is the fundamental essence of everything. At its highest, most pristine and sublime energetic state, this one energy is referred to as *Parama Shiva*. From this singular state, the one energy, out of its own free will and desire to experience itself and its bliss more, becomes two—***Shiva*** and ***Shakti***, the first two tattvas.

Shiva is considered masculine (although not male) in essence, and **Shakti** is considered feminine (although not female.) Shiva often corresponds to something known as *prakasha*, or the eternal light without which nothing can appear.

Shakti often corresponds to something known as *vimarsa*, the mirror upon which the reflection of Shiva's light is cast. Since we are apparently discussing two different aspects of the One, Shiva and Shakti cannot be fully separated. They are reliant upon one another, just as light and heat are different aspects of the same fire. They are the two tools that Param Shiva uses to know itself more deeply and to delight in its own exquisite joy.

Param Shiva, out of its own free will, first becomes Shiva-Shakti, and further divides itself into three main aspects (tattvas): **divine will, divine knowledge** and **divine action**. For the purposes of simplicity I have chosen to refer to these aspects in English rather than Sanskrit.

At this point the Divine and its first five manifestations is still in its fullness in what is known as the absolute realm, and its true nature is not bound or cloaked by ***maya,*** Sanskrit for "that which measures." The tattva maya is that which makes experience measurable or limited. It is that which separates and excludes things from one another. In the traditions of Kashmir Shaivism, maya is seen as that which begins a contraction or limitation. Maya draws a veil on supreme consciousness, on divine grace, or the Highest. As a result, the self in the manifest world forgets its real nature.

Maya generates a sense of difference among all things. For us humans, maya is a consequence of embodiment, as all energy manifesting in the relative world is subject to the conditions of maya.

Prior to physical manifestation, in what we call the psychical realm, the Divine manifests under one or more of five coverings—we call these the conditions or products of maya. These coverings act as limits on the full, undifferentiated and unlimited aspects of the Divine: (Shiva-Shakti, divine will, divine knowledge and divine action.) The coverings (five tattvas) are:

- The cloak over the divine action, which limits agency and doership,
- The cloak over divine knowledge, which limits knowledge,
- The cloak over the divine will, which limits satisfaction and creates longing,
- The cloak of Shakti, which reduces the freedom and pervasiveness of the universal consciousness and brings about limitation in respect to cause, space and form.
- The cloak of Shiva, which reduces time and creates past present and future.

The Divine, or essential energy of life, now cloaked and limited, enters the manifest world or the relative realm, where Shiva-Shakti becomes spirit and nature, respectively. Shiva is spirit, also known as ***purusha***, through the power of maya, which limits universal knowledge, and becomes the individual subject or soul. Shakti is nature, also called ***prakriti***, through the power of maya, and is the matrix of all of creation. Nature is necessary for spirit to have agency and the power to act.

Nature has three *gunas* or genetic constituents: *sattva guna*, *rajo guna* and *tamo guna*. In her unmanifest state, nature holds these gunas in perfect equipoise. Just as spirit and nature are the microcosmic reflections of Shiva and Shakti, the gunas are the microcosmic reflection of divine knowledge, divine will and divine action.

Sattva guna is characterized in the order of being by brightness and lightness. In the psychological domain, sattva guna expresses itself as transparency, joy and peace. In the ethical order, sattva guna is the principle of goodness. Sattva guna is responsible for lightheartendess, clear thought and happiness.

Rajo guna is characterized in the order of being by craving and passion. Rajo guna is associated with jealousy, anger and greed in the psychological domain. In the ethical order, rajas guna is the principle of ambition and avarice. Rajas is also the power of activity, of motivation, or will and energy. Through rajas guna we create and accomplish; it is the source of our will power.

Tamo guna is characterized by the principle of darkness and inertness in the order of being. Psychologically, tamo guna is marked by dullness, delusion and dejection. In the ethical order, it is the principle of degradation, debasement. Through tamo guna we are steadfast, patient, reliable and enduring.

Nature differentiates itself further into the psychic apparatus, the senses and matter. The psychic apparatus, or the inner instrument, consists of three tattvas called intuitive intelligence, the I-maker, and the mind.

The **intuitive intelligence** *(buddhi)* is just that—intuitively intelligent. It is the aspect of the psyche that is discriminating, pure, and closest to our divine source. The **I-maker** (*Ahamkara*) is its byproduct, and creates a sense of differentiation and separateness. The byproduct of the I-maker is the **mind**, (manas) which cooperates with the senses to build our perceptions. Interestingly, mind even has its own capacity to generate images and concepts, much like the I-maker.

Additional tattvas, other tools of the I-maker, are the powers of sense perception: **smelling, tasting, seeing, feeling by touch**, and **hearing**.

More gross in energy are the tattvas called the **powers of action: speaking, handling, locomotion, excreting,** and **sexual action**. Also categorized are the general elements of the particulars of sense perception: **sound, touch, color, flavor**, and **odor**.

Finally, the tattvas of materiality are the last classified. These are the five elements: **space, air, fire, water**, and **earth** which make up everything in the manifest world.(3)

The Great Game

According to these philosophies, "the human dilemma" is our experience of separation and differentiation from the Divine. This apparent state of separation is the result of a contraction or cloaking that occurs as the Highest moves through these stages from supreme undifferentiated energy into the world of differentiated form and matter. Revelation, or the yogic task, is to recognize the original state of union whereby we know the underlying consciousness that informs all of manifestation and realize that we are a part of that supreme consciousness.

Yoga is the means by which we begin to climb back up through the stages that the Supreme has traveled, gaining mastery and understanding of the various levels of consciousness and manifestation. Similar to a great game of hide and seek, the one energy of the Divine hides from itself in various ways for the sheer thrill of rediscovering itself and enjoying the reunion.(5) The spiritual practitioner, then, through yogic practices and with the assistance of the Highest, endeavors to find the Divine in its many guises and hiding places.

Understanding the various levels and manifestations of spirit is one way we can learn about the Supreme's hiding places. Knowing the places where the Divine is hiding can help us play the hide and seek game more skillfully. We can learn how best to apply our efforts in sadhana so that we increase the likelihood of discovering the ways our true nature is concealed and hidden from our awareness, of finding the joy and freedom of our truest self over and over again, throughout life's varied experiences and challenges.

For instance, this overview of the tattvas (again, refer to the schematic in the Appendix) teaches us that our consciousness, sometimes called the *antahkarana*—or the psychic or inner vehicle—is made up of three parts: the *buddhi*, the *ahamkara* and the *manas*. The highest aspect is considered the buddhi, the intuitive, discriminative mind. Under that is the ahamkara, the sense of I or me that makes up our identity and sense of self. These levels are then informed by the manas—that aspect of mind that gathers information through the senses and the organs of action. In order to climb the implicit order back up, to gain access to the buddhi, we must pass through the world of the senses and the world of the personality that defines our sense of self. If our senses are continually ingesting toxins, be they gross or subtle, the ahamkara and the buddhi are affected negatively and perpetuate our perception of being separate from our Divine essence. Conversely, our dharmic choices to ingest beauty, purity, and life-enhancing food through our senses will predispose the ahamkara toward a positive resonance with the buddhi, its wisdom and innate beauty.

Even if we choose to act out of alignment with these teachings, we can do so from a level of informed choice, rather than ignorance. We see that aligning with the Highest, when based on the dharma, can have a quality of an almost scientific approach. Putting the Highest first and creating strong walls of support is not in any way haphazard or arbitrary, but rather, follows an orderly set of principles that are found throughout nature.

Questions to Consider and Write About

1. What does dharma mean to you?
2. In what ways does philosophical understanding assist you in making optimal choices in your sadhana?
3. What areas of your life might benefit from some dharmic "walls of support"?

twelve

Spiritual Authority and the Guru

The Guru is the grace-bestowing power of the Supreme.
—Shiva Sutra Vimarshini

I frequently reflect on the irony that, while often yoga attracts very liberally-minded people who, in many cases, have had a falling out with traditional forms of religion, the foundation of yoga practice is a conservative tradition with fairly strict suggestions for appropriate conduct.

Yoga initially became popular in the West in the 1960s and 1970s during a time of free-wheeling consciousness exploration that was divorced from traditional ethics, morality and organized religion. In many cases, yoga still attracts people who like to think for themselves and who cherish ideals like individuality and autonomy, over and above the ideals of obedience and discipleship found throughout the history and traditions of yoga. This in and of itself is not a problem. In fact we must remember that many great innovations—even in the practice of yoga—were at one point in time seen as radical or in opposition to traditional viewpoints and ideas.

Interestingly, one of the most common expressions I hear in the workshops and classes I teach is "my yoga." Usually people say this when sharing about their beliefs, ideas and interpretations of yogic principles. Many times people say "It's my yoga" but mean, "Therefore I do it *my way*." And while I believe that each one of us does have "our yoga" to do, our unique personal journey of exploration and service, my experience is that the current trends in yoga do not give adequate voice to the power of self-deception along the way that traditional core practices have always sought to confront.

In my experience, we can learn from authoritative sources what *yoga is*, while we are exploring what *our yoga is*. My sincere wish is that we all avail ourselves of the help that the tradition has for us, and that experienced guides have for us, *before* we craft our own way through this demanding spiritual journey called *yoga*. By rooting ourselves in tradition and getting guidance from reliable teachers, our personal expression of yoga is developed relative to the tradition of yoga, and our personal synthesis is informed by an authoritative lineage, instead of being dictated by our ego-centric personal ideas, opinions and assumptions.

I asked my philosophy teacher Carlos Pomeda about what he considered "reliable sources." He answered me by first explaining the concept of spiritual authority:

> By "spiritual authority" I mean that the teachings and practices someone promulgates originate from "certain" (i.e., solid) knowledge, from experience rather than speculation or mere intellectual understanding. As you know, the tradition has always marked two kinds of knowledge (often using the terms *jnana* and *vijnana* to differentiate them): intellectual knowledge or book learning, and experiential wisdom. There's obviously nothing wrong with the first one, but it clearly is not enough ... The long and short of it is that only someone

> who has direct experience has the strong "authority" that is necessary in the teaching of yoga.
>
> There's a sliding scale, depending on what is at stake. For example, if I want to teach certain concepts of, say, Vedanta, and I make a small factual mistake, there's probably no great harm done. If I'm teaching asana, however, I better know how to guide people and give them the "inside" scoop on how to move forward. But if we're talking about deeper aspects of meditation, such as *kundalini* or the *cakras*, and I'm doing so without real direct experience, the consequences can be disastrous not only physically but mentally, emotionally and spiritually. It's not only the problem of misleading people or passing on worthless speculation, but the very real possibility of actual harm that is at stake.(1)

He continued by discussing the qualifications of a teacher from whom one would accept education in what yoga is and how to practice it:

> The yoga tradition has always set up parameters. For example, if a seeker wanted to accept someone as their guru, the traditional guidelines are at least three-fold: the person has to be enlightened, knowledgeable and authorized. That means:
>
> a. Enlightened. They've reached the "end of the road" so that they can speak with the authority we discussed in the earlier paragraph, so that they can have the deep insight required to offer proper guidance and so that they can transmit that same experience to others.

b. Knowledgeable. It's not enough to have the experience; they also need the "skills" to be a successful guide for others. They need to be able to offer a framework that will support their students' practice and they need to be able to understand the wide variety of experiences that their students will undergo. This is not possible without deep, extensive preparation.

c. Just like no one would decide to give themselves a Ph.D., no one can make themselves a guru (or worse, an "avatar" or such other claim!) without having been anointed by their own guru. While it is true that a few great beings have attained their state without external guidance, these are, in fact, the minority that confirms the rule.

So, how does this translate to our present situation? Well, I think at the very least students should become savvy enough to ask a few questions: What is the person's "pedigree"? Who was/were their teacher/s? How long have they trained? How much have they practiced and how deeply? Most importantly, what is their level of inner experience? Have they dived into the depths of their own being? What have they learned? How much have they studied? How much experience do they have in guiding others? Finally, how do they live? Do their lives reflect their beliefs and teachings, or do they say one thing and do something completely different? Are they happy, fulfilled individuals? And so on . . .[2]

Additionally, I asked Mr. Pomeda about resistance in practice, knowing that even with a great teacher and a willing, open heart, sadhana is difficult, and that giving up "our way" and taking guidance in "the Way" is often quite challenging. He remarked:

> Resistance is part of the process; it goes with the territory. In traditional India, the idea was that you would test a guru thoroughly before accepting them (this is what my paramaguru Baba Muktananda used to say) because once you're through with the testing, the guru will begin to test you! In other words, you wanted to be very, very, very clear that you didn't just have blind faith on someone because the inner journey is not always easy and one is tested every step of the way.
>
> In our present day, however, I don't think this type of attitude translates well. Certainly in the West we don't have the same tradition of "surrender" or acceptance of authority; quite the opposite! Clearly, there are plusses and minuses to both types of attitudes, but the bottom line is that one needs trust in any teaching/learning situation. As long as one is resistant, no change is possible. And while one should never relinquish discrimination (quite the opposite), one needs first of all the introspection to identify and examine resistance as well as the willingness to take a bold step forward every now and then. Ultimately, I believe it's the burning desire for enlightenment that helps one move beyond all barriers, resistance included.(3)

Having a teacher is essential to learning and growing on the path of yoga. On the simplest level, just practicing the yoga asanas requires a skill set that few of us know intrinsically. How, without a teacher, will we really learn the poses, the requisite actions and the necessary refinements?

Even though the yogic path essentially points us to our inner teacher and to our own innate wisdom, proper guidance is required to navigate the journey. Practicing yoga and building a temple of the body involves entering uncharted territory and facing obstacles with which we have no prior experience. Availing ourselves of the help of an experienced guide is simply a wise course of action to take in such a circumstance.

Most of us can look back over our lives and list people whose influence has been instrumental in making us who we are today. Teachers cultivate our talents, help us hone our skills, point out our blind spots and assist us in shedding those habits that block us from our deepest truths.

The Guru

In Sanskrit the word for teacher is *guru*. It means "heavy, authoritative, and/or weighty," as in someone who has the weight of spiritual authority. It can also be understood by looking to the clues that the word itself provides. The word guru is made up of two parts: *gu*- meaning darkness and -*ru* meaning light. The guru, then is "that which brings light to darkness." The guru is best understood as a function, rather than a person. The guru, at its conceptual essence, is a function of the Highest that manifests through certain people or circumstances in order to reveal to us our true nature and the nature of reality. The guru exists to remind us that everything is Supreme Consciousness and to help us find what is hidden in the great hide-and-seek game of Reality. In a general way, good teachers become the agents of the guru function, bringing light to our darkness and showing us who we most truly are.

Occasionally, the guru function becomes extremely potent in certain individuals, as though they are a condensed and established source of the Highest's revelatory power. These rare individuals earn the title of *sadguru*, which means "the true guru" or "teacher of the Real." More than an ordinary teacher, the sadguru is "celebrated as a potent agent of Grace."(4) The sadguru's responsibility is to guide a disciple toward a complete recognition of the nature of reality itself, not simply to assist a student in a yoga pose or facilitate flashes of insight.

In the case of a sadguru, the guru function works as much by a process of entrainment and resonance as it does by any linear teaching methodology. For instance, my yoga teacher, John Friend, often talks about how if you put little clocks in the same room with a big grandfather clock, after a period of time the small clocks will begin to work in sync with the larger clock. That phenomenon of synching up with the big clock is known as entrainment. This process of entrainment is at the heart of the guru-disciple relationship, wherein the student, through a process of education, practice and in many cases physical and/or energetic proximity, develops a resonance to the influence of the Highest that is manifesting through his or her teacher.

It is this force, manifesting through the teacher, that my guru suggests is the real transformational agent in the process of waking up. He said:

> Well, in the real sense it's not *sadhana* that produces awakening. It's assimilation that produces awakening. So to assimilate something, you have to be in its field, in its aura. The guru is that which is grace, living grace, and the real essence of *sadhana* is to assimilate that. When the disciple wakes up, it's because they've assimilated the guru's Grace, not because they've done *sadhana*. Paradoxically, one has to do *sadhana* to create the kind of resonance that allows the assimilation to occur. *Sadhana* is like preparing the field, but really it is all grace. And to get grace, you have to be in relationship to grace. You don't have to be in its physical presence necessarily, although there are benefits to that. You can get it anywhere as long as

> you hook into it. But the guru is the hook, the source of it.(5)

Obviously, stories abound about gurus who have exploited their students' trust and who have misused their power and authority. Volumes have been written refuting the claim that a teacher is necessary in any way. (Arguing those points is not only outside the scope of this book, it is outside the scope of my interest.) In every subject matter pursued there are good teachers and poor teachers. In every discipline there are teachers who effectively communicate their expertise and clarity to their students and those teachers who fail miserably. And just as there are good and bad teachers, so too does the skill of the student vary greatly from circumstance to circumstance.

At the heart of most debate regarding gurus is a lack of proper understanding about the true nature of the guru-disciple relationship. Issues of power, authority and obedience strike at the core of our Western ideals of independence and free thought. Others find it quite objectionable that a person would seemingly be "worshipped" in a way that is typically reserved only for God. Even simple gestures like bowing down in front of a guru, for instance, are so far outside our cultural norms that the ritual of bowing in offering and obedience is not seen in the appropriate context. Pictures of spiritual teachers, statues of gurus and other spiritual paraphernalia seem to make people nervous and skeptical of the whole idea all together. On the surface, out of context and without proper education, these outer manifestations of the guru-disciple relationship are understandably confusing at best and, more often than not, frightening or off-putting.

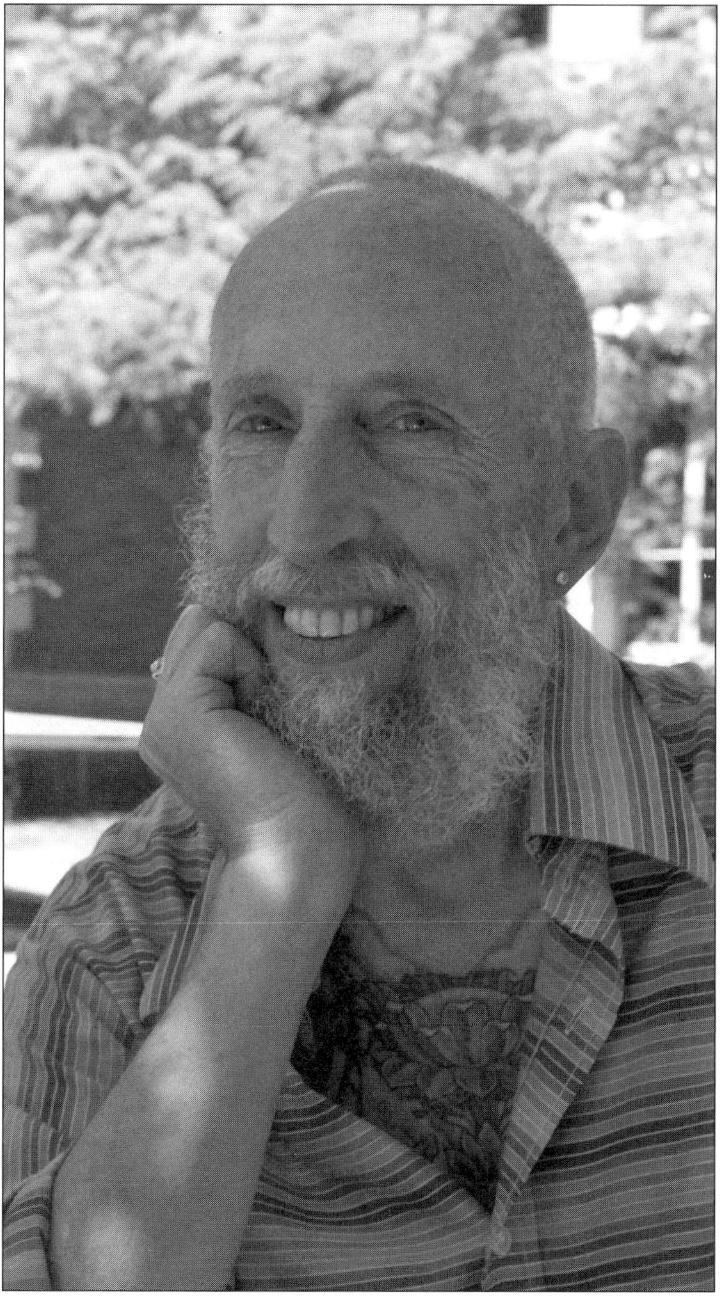

Lee Lozowick

Interestingly, those of us involved in a traditional relationship with a guru have no trouble seeing other traditions, like Christianity, in those exact terms. Yet most Christians probably find the notion of a guru quite distasteful and even heretical. My view is that Jesus was a great teacher who brought light to darkness and whose spiritual influence may very well be unparalleled. According to all stories about Jesus, he functioned exactly like any guru from the yoga traditions. (In fact, he is considered by many in the Hindu faith to have been a great yogi!) My point is simply that the unfamiliar traditions and terminology that often go along with gurus seem to create a skepticism that is, in my opinion, largely unwarranted.

Additionally, far too many people worry about the trustworthiness of various gurus without examining and being responsible for their own reliability, discernment and clarity as students or devotees. Truly, it is rare that anyone is exploited by a guru without his or her own consent. To be a worthy disciple we must be clear about the motives, expectations and projections that we are placing on any spiritual authority figure. One must place trust and faith carefully, and gradually.

My guru says:

> Superficially, it is very hard to tell who is a real Teacher. Anyone can act and imitate being a spiritual Teacher, so the student has to look deeper. What you'll always find is one who is kind, generous with his or her time and resources, who is soft and heartful and displays a full range of emotional expression. If he is a man and he can't cry, he is not a real Master. But paradoxically, a real Teacher will surely work in a way to be misunderstood and generate animosity if that will serve his students.[6]

Testimony

Personally, I wouldn't want to approach the task of sadhana without the assistance and guidance of a guru. I cherish and rely on my guru's help. He has served as a tangible agent of the Highest and a source of wisdom, clarity and blessings that have helped me in countless ways since I have been in his company. For me, our relationship is indispensable, as he is the way that I have been able to directly experience many of the teachings of yoga that for years eluded me. Prior to my relationship with Lee Lozowick, the Highest was more of an idea, rather than a direct experience.

John Friend points to this idea of grace being a direct experience in this description of his first meeting with his guru, Gurumayi Chidvalasananda:

> When I felt Her Presence, I felt a real, tangible presence that was apparently emanating from her but was moving within me and it was able to make great shifts within my body, mind and spirit. Then I learned to soften and attune to that energy more, instead of hardening. What I used to do is just try to do it by myself so I ended up just being harder. But when I tuned into the energy by softening, I was able to do a lot more and it came from not only being more sensitive but by respecting myself more and having self-love.
>
> She guided me like that. She was strong enough—her energy was strong enough—that I literally felt it inside. It was something! I never felt like that before . . . It was really Real.(7)

While I believe that having a yoga teacher it essential, I do not believe that everybody who practices hatha yoga needs to be involved in a traditional guru-disciple relationship. For instance, a knowledgeable hatha yoga teacher can assist her students in learning the postures safely and practicing pranayama effectively, and will almost always be a source of inspiration for her students on and off the yoga mat. I do not believe that a traditional guru-disciple relationship is necessary to live a good and meaningful life or to make progress on the Path. Scores of people serve tirelessly and realize their dreams and deep spiritual longings without a guru. However, I do believe that the guru as a function is inescapable, because the guru function is part of the revelatory aspect of the Highest. As such, the guru function is simply one way that the Highest expresses itself.

Guru and Grace

According to the traditions of Kashmir Shaivism, there are five main ways that the Divine expresses itself or "acts" in an ultimate sense. Stated another way, there are five functions of grace. Grace creates, sustains, destroys, conceals and reveals. The revelatory aspect of grace is called *anugraha*, which has the root "*graha*" meaning "to grab." Anugraha is that aspect of grace that grabs hold of us, supports us and does for us what we cannot do for ourselves. The revelation of grace is considered to be something outside of our own effort. Anugraha does not discount those things that we can and should be responsible for in our journey of awakening, it simply recognizes that there is a job to be done that requires a kind of support outside the domain of our own self-effort.

As the revelatory aspect of grace, the guru function expresses itself along a continuum of forms: from potent yet ordinary experiences that help us glimpse deeper truths of the heart (like watching an inspirational sunset); to good teachers who serve and uplift their immediate sphere of influence;

to spiritual heavyweights whose work and skillful means far exceed just being a good teacher, but is focused on a more universal mission.

Different Ways to Relate

How different people relate to the guru function will most certainly vary greatly, because just as the guru function expresses itself over a continuum, so does the function of studentship. Each one of us is called to a unique expression of studentship and devotion to these ideals. Some students on the yoga path will serve a teacher directly, others will serve more peripherally. Some students will live a life of renunciation and strict adherence to the practices of a sect or particular tradition. Some students of yoga will have no inclination toward formal involvement in organized religious traditions but will uplift and inspire others and work for positive change in the world quite heroically. Some studentship will express itself as conscious parenting. The list of the ways that studentship might manifest is long and varied.

In what ways can you make use of the teachers in your life? This is a question relevant to the task of building a temple of the body through yoga, not about whether or not one needs a traditional guru. In what ways can we, as students, become increasingly skillful so that the guru function supports and upholds our practice and our desire to become a great temple of divine inspiration? For instance, if we have a traditional guru, in what ways can we move into greater resonance? Whether or not we have a formal relationship with a guru, we must continually ask ourselves if we are allowing ourselves to be instructed by life itself. Are we cultivating receptivity to life that is beyond the confines of our own opinions, preferences and projections?

We Are Not Separate

> While we know that it is imperative that once you decided to take Bhagwan as your master, there could never be a question of deciding whether or not you liked certain things about His life—it was still difficult to practice this so that it naturally came into play. The mind is always looking for a way to separate and divide, to count and measure, when what truly matters is much more quietly burning in the heart. When you accepted Yogi Ramsuratkumar as your master, you had to abide by whatever he said. Your pleasure, your willingness or unwillingness, your desire, don't exist at all when His command comes. Total faith demands this. To be of service to the master demands this. —Mani, *A Man and His Master*, 115.

The guru, in all of its forms, and the student are inextricably bound in the process of awakening called yoga. Even the best teacher will be limited in his or her influence if the student is not prepared adequately to make use of him or her. When, as students, we are committed to our own preparation process, our own adhikara, we begin, more and more, to free the teacher to actually teach us. Lee Lozowick has often said that in the beginning of the relationship the guru's grace will carry the student. But after a while it is only lawful that students learn to walk by themselves. Once that level of care is no longer required of the guru, the guru can apply his or her attention to the deeper aspects of the transformational process such as assisting the student in refining their sadhana by directing the student's efforts more effectively.

As students we must take the generosity of our teacher's grace that has carried us and use it to bolster ourselves so that we become able to generate our own esteem, our own confidence and our own capacity for self-love. When we do this—when the positive self-regard becomes our own and becomes implicit in the relationship with our teacher—then the level of support the teacher is able to give takes a quantum leap. Essentially, the guru is not an outer support mechanism, but that which instructs us in how to support and stabilize ourselves; a true guru or teacher is one whose light helps us discover our own light.

Questions to Consider and Write About

1. In what way is the guru function alive in your life?
2. In what ways have you experienced the bestowal of grace or anugraha?
3. In what ways might you bolster your studentship?
4. Who in your life has been a vehicle of the guru function? This might be a child, a friend, a relative, a teacher, a spiritual guide or a traditional guru.

thirteen

The Kula

You become the company you keep, so keep great company.

—Swami Baba Muktananda

Call it a clan, call it a network, call it a tribe, call it a family. Whatever you call it, whoever you are, you need one.

—Jane Howard

Kula is a Sanskrit word that means family or clan. Family, in this case, refers to one's family of spiritual practitioners or one's spiritual community. Spiritual community is a specific type of community that operates according to different rules and obligations than social communities. Spiritual community, for instance, does not imply that we all agree on matters of politics, nutrition, finances and fashion, or even that we like each other and enjoy one another's personalities all the time. Kula, after all, does not mean clique or social network. A kula is that group of people who decide to come together, who find communion together in the practice of yoga and who choose to uphold similar virtues of the heart. The context of kula is decidedly outside the domain of mundane affairs and concerns.

Having a group of people with whom to practice yoga and with whom to share the journey of awakening is another support structure for the temple of the body. I know firsthand the transformational aspect of community. In the beginning of my personal process of making peace with my body, I was dangerously wrapped up in my own distorted views of beauty and physical appearances. Having a group of people who were dedicated to helping me grow spiritually was necessary in order to shift my external focus on appearances to an internal focus of growth, surrender and spiritual practice.

On a recent visit to my teacher's ashram, I was helping my friend set the table for dinner. I noticed that I felt happy and relaxed. The quality of relaxation I felt was distinctly different from that of my usual relaxing at the end of the day. I realized that I had truly let down my psychic/psychological guard—a barrier that I didn't even know I had up! In the company of people who knew me, who valued my inner life and my being more than they value my appearance or my professional credentials, I found a refuge in which I could relax and experience a different aspect of myself than I normally do.

The more we experience this type of refuge, and the more we come to experience who we are in these moments of letting our guard down, I believe we will come to prefer the state of being that arises in the company of the kula over and above the company of strictly social relationships. Instead of finding the world of outer appearances and shallow social concerns and connections so captivating, we will seek out the company of the real. And in the company of the real, in the refuge of those who have our highest purposes in mind, we will be more likely to align our outer behaviors and our attitude with the deeper truths of our heart.

Strength in Making Changes

In building a temple of the body we may be making changes in our outer behaviors. We may realize that a life of excess and indulgence is counter to our yogic purposes, and yet we may find that establishing ourselves in a new way is difficult. The kula is an invaluable source of support in helping to ground ourselves in discipline and practice. For instance, after many years of regularly attending the morning meditation practice on my teacher's ashram, I had stopped going and had fallen off the wagon. I had gotten swept up into the demands of my life and dropped this practice from my priorities. After a while, I missed the influence of meditation and I really wanted to go back. I would swear to myself every night that "tomorrow I will get up and go." And yet, the next morning would come and I would sleep in and make excuses for myself. I realized that I needed support in this situation.

So, I called one of my friends and made a verbal commitment to her that I would be in the meditation hall in the mornings. I then asked several of my kula mates whom I knew went to meditation regularly to help me uphold my commitment to practice. I asked several people to phone me if they noticed I had missed several days and just invite me back to meditation. It worked. Having people to hold me accountable to my commitment to practice helped me strengthen my resolve to practice. The kula held me up until I was strong enough to get to meditation without the help of the external support structure.

Kula or community also gives us an opportunity to see ourselves in the context of relationship. Often, a relationship with someone highlights our pockets of insecurity, fear and tendency for manipulation. Sometimes, in the context of relationship, we see aspects of ourselves that do not show up when we are alone. And, while the knowledge of our true colors is not always easy to see or to accept, clarity about these blind spots is ultimately one of the great gifts that community offers.

Practicing in a group demands that we compromise, communicate clearly, and rub up against one another's personalities and idiosyncratic behaviors. In the friction of interpersonal dynamics we see areas of self that we need to work on, and the ways we might benefit from psychological purification and increased maturity. Imagine being in a yoga class when the person next to you has practiced Darth Vader-like *ujayi pranayama* all the way through *savasana* and you have felt like screaming in frustration. Perhaps you did not think you had a lot of anger, and yet, on this occasion you were about to tear your hair out if that person took just one more deep breath! And most of us, if we are honest, will admit to having experienced something similar at one point or another. That frustration, that view of ourselves in a moment of interpersonal reactivity, invites us into a deeper level of personal practice and accountability.

The frustrations we find in relationship and in functioning as part of a group are not signs that the *community* is "off" or that practicing within a community is not useful. Rather, these difficulties are signs that the group work is indeed working; that who we are is being revealed in greater fullness. For many years Lee Lozowick has stated that he can best be understood within the context of community. He continually suggests that our ability or inability to function as part of a group is a sign of progress (or lack thereof) on the Path. Considering this deeply we see that at the heart of the Path is the affirmation of strength through unity, and the invitation to invest in another's progress on the Path as well as our own.

From I to We

Shifting our emphasis from a strictly self-centered approach to a unified community-based approach is an opportunity to confront our deeply held beliefs of separation, isolation and competition. Greatness, success and accomplishment need not be limited or achieved only at the expense of someone else.

Rather, this model of community asks each of us to dedicate attention and intention to one another, not at the expense of our own practice, but as an adjunct to it. Thus, we learn to be as interested in someone else's greatness as we are in our own. Instead of life and/or sadhana being an ongoing game of one-upmanship where only one person can win, we dedicate ourselves to the ideal that our success is relative, that is, in relationship to the success of one another.

This points us to the ideal that the purpose of practice in the context of a *kula* is serving the highest in one another. This is our common aim. Obviously, such an ideal is not realized easily or without personality conflicts. In aiming high, after all, we may often miss the mark. But in the aiming, the missing, the re-adjusting and the repeated attempts, our skill in yoga is cultivated. Building a temple of the body is a yoga of inclusion and teamwork, where the support of the kula is regarded as paramount. Refining ourselves in relationship to such a vision is certainly a worthwhile aim.

Many examples of teamwork aligned with a common aim can be found in the narrative of Yogi Ramsuratkumar's temple-building project. Over time, the workers on this temple became a kula. They were no longer doing a construction job merely for money; they were no longer concerned only about their personal needs and wishes. Instead, they were working in service to a spiritual master and his wishes. Throughout the course of the project they continually deepened their alignment and reliance on Yogi Ramsuratkumar's force of blessing in order to get their jobs done. As Mani, the project manager, wrote: "There were at the busiest time of construction, over four hundred workers—masons, bar benders, shuttering laborers, dome fabricators, carpenters, men and women laborers of all levels of skill. These people worked together as a group without problems, without excessive noise; everyone treated the work at hand as divine work."(1)

Simply put, the teamwork was possible because the workers had a common aim and understood that grace was the source of the work.

Blessed Work

There was a natural development of workers bringing their raw materials and hand tools to Bhagwan for blessing—trowels, shovels, buckets, cement trays and welding rods—to be blessed by Him. They knew that the power of this building project was sitting before them and if His blessings were invoked, there would be success. They had witnessed enough to know that it was not their handiwork alone that was making this building. If He touched the materials or tools, the responsibility of the building became His Father's work. He imbued His Father's divine blessing into every material that passes into His beautiful buildings.

He fed us His prasad, purifying us to work with the blessed tools and materials. On some level we could feel the sacredness of our work with Him. The awareness of this was so deep within that it seemed to be at an unconscious level. The expression of what we were constructing at this deep level was an extension of Yogi Ramsuratkumar, built for the benefit of devotees, spiritual seekers and the unity of the world. —Mani, *A Man and His Master*, 178.

Time and again the workers on Yogi Ramsuratkumar's ashram did the impossible because they were united in a common aim of serving him. United under a common aim and guided by an agent of grace, the power of the worker-kula became greater than that of any one person. They accomplished as a bonded group what people acting as individuals would never have been able to realize. This is the value of group practice.

To build a temple of our body, we too have the support of the kula. To utilize this supportive structure, we must continually align ourselves with grace within the context of community. The support of the community will actually be proportional to our willingness to serve the community and to serve within the parameters of a group. Over time we will realize that by serving one another we are, ourselves, being served.

The Team Effort

The element of teamwork to execute this work flawlessly, without accident was impressive. Despite the intensity of the pace to move wet concrete, the degree of difficulty in accomplishing this work without machines and the dangers of the construction zone, this work went on without incident. There were gas-powered cement mixers, frequently repeated infusions of gas poured into the fuel tanks, heavy loads of concrete changing many hands at unsecured heights, trucks backing in and driving out while a little over a hundred people accomplished in a day what would have required millions of dollars worth of machinery to do elsewhere. Workers were barefoot, without hard

> hats and sunscreen, no red-flagged danger zones, but every laborer possessing a keen sense of awareness of basic safety and common sense in working around such dangers. As if Bhagwan was the conductor in a great orchestra, each worker moved with a sense of timing that used no more or less energy than necessary to complete the task at their post. They followed His meticulous attention to the construction as if in slow motion to avoid mishap and accident. At full speed, however, the pace was furious. Everyone seemed to be yelling different directions simultaneously and at high volume but all effort was in the team movement of cement and not in attention to whatever was being said.—Mani, *A Man and His Master*, 173.

Lee Lozowick once used the analogy that a spiritual community is like a soup. He told one of his students who was having doubts about how she contributed positively to the community that she had to think of herself as a bay leaf. Alone, a bay leaf appears to be just a little dried up leaf. But when added to the soup, that bay leaf imparts a delicious flavor that becomes an essential ingredient in the recipe. Each one of us in the kula is like that bay leaf. We have our unique attributes and characteristics, but our true purpose is not realized until those attributes are dedicated to the whole; until we dedicate our own uniqueness to "making the soup fantastic."(2)

More Personal Testimony

Being part of "making the soup fantastic," over and above being a great single ingredient, is the invitation of the kula. This idea can be found across traditions. For instance, my parents have always been active members of The United Methodist Church and for many years my father has talked with me about one of the attributes of his faith called "The Community of Believers." After he read my book *Yoga from the Inside Out*, he told me that much of what I had written about community echoed his experience within the Christian Community of Believers:

> The Community of Believers within the Judeo-Christian faith tradition exists to profess, proclaim, witness to, and serve the risen Christ through ministry to our brothers and sisters. For those of us already within this faith, the community nourishes us, informs us, facilitates our interaction with God, and teaches us how to live. Because of the joy and meaning we find within the community, we wish to bring others to the group, without, as may be inferred from the above, any coercion or "preaching" of condemnation for those outside that community.(3)

My father shared with me about his own spiritual development relative to the idea of community:

> As you know, I was born into, and raised in, the Judeo-Christian tradition, specifically the Presbyterian Church . . . In a typical but exaggerated Jungian-type experience, I early became focused on individuation, in large part due to the family situation in which I was enmeshed. This personal individuation resulted in my discounting, or rather, not understanding the importance of community for many years. That is, I had an individualistic outlook on life in general and the church in particular.

> Jungians might suggest that my "return" to community is the result of natural progression. Over time, I became aware of the comfort of being within a community as opposed to trying to make my life journey alone. In any event, I profess that the Community of Believers has become paramount for me.[(4)]

Even in this brief account of a lifetime of practice within the church, my father's sharing points out the kind of opening that can happen for any of us when we recognize that we are supported by others of like heart and mind, and when we allow ourselves to find comfort in that support. We recognize that we are not alone. In practicing together, in dedicating ourselves to one another's highest potential, we become a body of people who, in sharing the same heart, also support and uphold one another like walls support and uphold any building.

Questions to Consider and Write About

1. In what ways does your kula support and uphold you?
2. What is currently challenging for you about community?

fourteen

Enthusiastic Discipline

Great Faith.
Great Doubt.
Great Effort.

The Three Qualities Necessary for Training
—*The Little Zen Companion*

Enthusiastic discipline is that discipline, or those acts of discipleship, that help us hold to the remembrance that God is within us. Great insight into the nature of enthusiastic discipline can be found in studying these two words and their etymologies. For instance, the word "enthusiasm" is composed of the prefix *en-* for "in" and the root *-theos* meaning "God." It is the state of being "possessed by God" or of "holding God within." "Discipline" comes from the same root as "disciple," which mean *to learn, to comprehend, to hold apart.* Discipline then, so often associated with great restraint and restriction can be understood as holding ourselves apart from behavior that interferes with learning and with comprehending. In this case what we are attempting to comprehend is the essence of who we are and what our true nature is.

No matter how inspiring the vision of building a temple of the body is, no matter how much we might want to align ourselves with the Highest, our sincere longing and inspirations must be brought to life through enthusiastic, disciplined efforts. These enthusiastic efforts will create the steadfast support necessary to build a strong and stable temple of the body that can weather any storm. While I believe that, in an absolute sense, the dharma, the guru and the kula are always present as supportive structures, in order for us to truly utilize them for support in our sadhana we must create behavior and attitudes that support us from the inside out. In cultivating our own internal support mechanisms, we become worthy of and able to access the support that comes through seemingly external sources.

We have already considered some of aspects of enthusiastic discipline in Chapter 8, *Adhikara*, when we looked at establishing our foundational attitude and lifestyle choices. Enthusiastic discipline is the ongoing mood of practice we must bring into building a temple of the body. Erecting a temple of the body, building it from the ground up, decorating it and worshipping within it is a vision worthy of enthusiasm. Its purpose is to help us become a vehicle able to hold God within, and to serve from that place or purpose.

Enthusiastic discipline is part of the scaffolding of our temple-building project, and its source is the wellspring of devotional longing within us. Enthusiastic discipline originates deep in the inner being of the practitioner. For instance, we are not holding ourselves apart from things we enjoy by some imposed restriction, but rather abstaining from those things that work against our highest aims and practicing those things that strengthen us, out of the recognition of what serves our deepest truths.

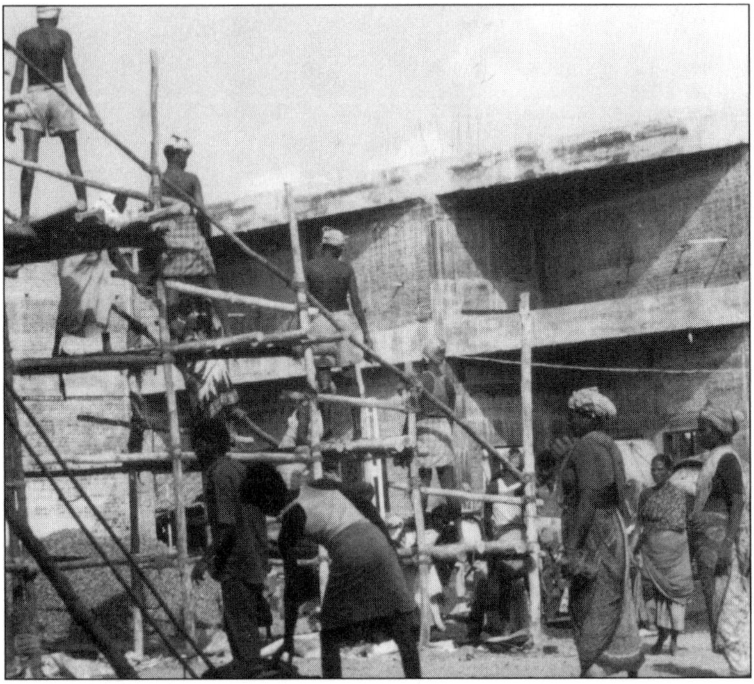

Both men and women labor in constructing the Temple of Yogi Ramsuratkumar, Tiruvannamalai, 1997.

Hard Work, Timing and Attention

The work was hard. The demands were constant. Mani was a powerful taskmaster, and Yogi Ramsuratkumar was, in his own way, harder. While assignments and scheduling varied, ashram staff were often expected to be available as early as five in the morning and to stay at their posts until eight at night, or later, depending upon the need. During one phase of the building, when both a day shift and a night shift were in operation, Mani himself was getting no more than two hours of sleep. When Raji [Mani's wife] became anxious for her husband's welfare, Yogi Ramsuratkumar took some time to assess her concern. Later, he spoke to her, clearly: "Father says two hours sleep is more than enough for Mani. Do not bother about it. My Father blesses you both."

Besides the expectation for simple hard work, timing and attention to detail had always been crucial to the Beggar. Nothing had really changed. Yet, now that he had an ashram to care for, Yogi Ramsuratkumar's expectations for this type of precision among his staff and attendants became even more obvious, as he was being seen and touched by more people. Teaching lessons on the subject came fast and furiously.

"I can be with somebody else and be casual about certain things," Saravanan, one of the ashram management team, began. "But with Him, if you are supposed to give coffee at 7:00 in the morning everyday, you should give it at 7:00 only. If you bring it at 6:45 A.M., he will never take it. He will wait until 7:00 A.M. to drink it, even if you give it at 6:45. If, the next day, you bring the coffee at 7:30, he will not drink coffee at all."

Yogi Ramsuratkumar never stopped working, with everyone. From the part-time day-laborer to his Eternal Slave, Devaki, his attention took the form of constant refinement. Time, energy, resources, money, lack of conflict . . . details . . . details . . . details. Everything was important to him.

"Once, when Ravi his driver took a holiday, I drove Bhagwan from Sudama House to the Ashram," Saravanan related, describing how the lesson in precision was delivered in his case. "One morning I went there a few minutes late, only five minutes. He was already sitting outside the gate on the stool. He just looked at me, as I slowly opened the door. I knew what it meant. Then, one year later, Ravi again took holiday. I went to Bhagwan to tell him that I would be his driver. 'Bhagwan, tomorrow morning I am coming at 6:45 A.M.,' I said. 'Don't come five minutes late,' Yogi Ramsuratkumar told me. He remembered exactly what had happened one year ago. So, I started coming thirty minutes early, just in case."—Regina Sara Ryan, *Only God, A Biography of Yogi Ramsuratkumar*, 554-555.

Tantra and Discipline

In my opinion, one of the more misunderstood aspects of tantra in the modern yoga milieu is in the area of discipline. I hear so many people who practice yoga using tantric scriptural references to justify behavior that is nothing other than undisciplined indulgence. For example, during the week that I taught about *bhoga* (enjoyment) and yoga merging on the path of the kula, an idea central to the *Kularnava Tantra*, I was disheartened to hear a group of my students reference this quote as rationale for their night of alcoholic excess.

Recently, at a yoga workshop, I went out to dinner after one of the sessions with a friend. Other participants, all of whom are longtime yoga practitioners and teachers were seated at another table across from us at the restaurant. After dinner, as my friend and I were leaving, we went to say good-bye to our friends at the other table. I looked down at their plates and at the table. Almost every person was eating meat and, among the six people seated, there were six open bottles of wine. I must have stared a bit or looked a little shocked, because one of the group made a comment about how it was "Okay because we are *tantrikas*."

I could go on about yoga "raves" and so-called "tantric parties"—that abound throughout the world of the pop-yoga scene—replete with drugs, alcohol and sexual play. I do not tell these stories to condemn the meat eaters in my readership. Nor am I preaching about abstinence from alcoholic beverages. Those who chose to use drugs—licit or illicit—have their reasons. These are personal choices. I do not claim to be a purist nor am I advocating a purist, renunciate lifestyle. Nonetheless, I have my opinions about the usefulness and dangers of mind- and mood-altering substances relative to yoga and conscious living, although I am not interested in arguing the subject here. I tell these stories to make the point that, while that meal or the night on the town or the "yoga rave" may have been a lot of things (enjoyable, tasty, yummy, fun, delicious, and exciting), they were not tantra in the sense of how those substances were traditionally incorporated into sadhana.

As modern practitioners of a traditionally-based path, we should not attempt to deceive ourselves or one another about such distinctions. The application of tantric principles and the ingesting of substances within tantric rituals are legitimately practiced only within the context of a highly disciplined lifestyle. Philosophically, the tantric traditions were as wide open and embracing as one could imagine, but practically speaking, that expansiveness stood on the firm ground of restraint, stability and maturity.

The *Kularnava Tantra* states:

> Wine to be drunk, flesh eaten and the fair face to be seen—this indeed is the object, this the way to be followed," many wrongly think. Deluded in

> themselves, bereft of the guidance of the Guru, they delude others too.
>
> If by mere drinking of wine one were to attain fulfillment, all drunkards would reach perfection.
>
> If mere partaking of flesh were to lead to the high estate, all flesh-eaters in the world would come by immense merit.
>
> If liberation were to ensue by mere cohabitation with woman, all creatures would stand liberated by female companionship.
>
> It is not the Kula Marga that is to be denounced, but those who do not tread it in the right spirit. One is the way that is laid down for the Kula from on high and quite other is the way followed by fools deeming themselves wise. You may walk on the sharp edge of a sword; you may hold on the sharp edge of a sword; you may wear a serpent on the body; but to follow aright the way of the Kula is much more difficult.
>
> ... It is only when things are processed through prescribed ritual and the partaker undergoes the prescribed self-modification, that the right results accrue.(1)

This text was written several centuries ago and from within a culture vastly different than that of twenty-first-century U.S.A. Obviously, not everything from tenth-century India will transfer to our times, and I appreciate that. I am simply urging all of us who subscribe to tantric ideals, in any way, to view these teachings with maturity, and to avoid twisting them to support those actions that might potentially take us further from our aim. While no thing is essentially bad, and while everything has the potential to be turned toward the path of the heart, whether or not that ideal is realized is a matter of skill. Skillful practice is cultivated through enthusiastic discipline and stands in stark contrast to anything motivated and explained by sentiments such as: "as much as I want," or "whatever I feel like," and "because I want to."

A Practice of Renunciation

At one point during that first year Yogi Ramsuratkumar asked Mani to engage an experiment. He said, "For one hundred days you stay on the ashram, you don't smoke, you don't drink alcohol, and you eat no meat or fish. You read no newspaper and watch no television. After one hundred days, then you can drink a quart of liquor if you want to."

It was a radical approach to a fast purification of his old lifestyle, and it worked. After the hundred days of abstinence, Mani went to Bhagwan exultant, "The one hundred days are over!" With Yogi Ramsuratkumar's blessing, he went out to a hotel with a friend to have the rich food, meat and whiskey he'd been dreaming of, but he was immediately surprised to find that it was all flat. He had no taste for it and didn't really want any of it. He knew that he would be unable to return to the fast life he used to lead.

When he returned to the ashram Yogi Ramsuratkumar asked, "How was it?"

"You know how it was!" Mani retorted humorously. Yogi Ramsuratkumar laughed and laughed. —M. Young, *Yogi Ramsuratkumar, Under the Punnai Tree*, 448.

Yes or No?

If we want to build a temple of the body, our behavior will either help us to construct a solid building or compromise the temple's structural integrity. In this somewhat black or white view of personal choices, there is no getting away with anything. Certainly we can try to pretend that our indulgence or our rigidity is just fine. In actuality, however, we are either building the temple of the body or we are condemning it.

Great self-honesty and great wisdom are required in order to discern what helps and what hurts, as each person and each situation is different. "Right" and "wrong" exist not as a set of rules that demand strict adherence, but in relationship to our ability to practice and dedicate ourselves to our chosen path reliably.

Enthusiastic discipline is the willingness to say yes and no appropriately, to give up those things—behavioral or attitudinal—that compromise our efforts so that we are able to hold God within. Consciously cultivating specific virtues, thoughts and actions strengthens us by drawing us in toward the core of our endeavor, to the heart of our aim, and away from the periphery of mundane distractions and concerns. When the scaffolding of the spirit is strong enough, and when it is maintained with enthusiastic discipline, we have a temple we can enter for worship, celebration and communion.

Questions to Consider and Write About

1. How does enthusiastic discipline apply to your relationship with your body?
2. How does enthusiastic discipline apply to your life of practice?
3. In what ways is your discipline enthusiastic?

PART IV

THE SANCTUARY: EXPANDING THE INNER LIFE OF THE TEMPLE

Having set our intention, laid the foundation and erected strong walls of support, we are now ready to cultivate the inner life of the temple and to expand our relationship with the source of spirit that lies in the heart of each of us.

fifteen

Beauty and the Expansion of the Inner Life

I looked in Temples, Churches and mosques.
I found the Divine in my heart.

—Rumi

In the asana practice, it is easy to stay preoccupied with the placement of our limbs, our posture, the alignment of our head (lift this, turn here, don't sag there, stay focused here, maintain this while you do that, put your hand here like this, not there like that). Truly, the work of perfecting the foundation and aligning one's outer posture is endless and fascinating. Even micro-movements can yield sometimes magnificent returns in any given pose, and the exploration of these relationships and outcomes within the body can be exhilarating, consuming, and even seductive and distracting, because the outer emphasis can direct our attention so one-pointedly to the *form* of the temple, that the *inner life* of the temple is neglected.

I have often discussed with seasoned yoga practitioners the merits of specific hand placement, technical details of alignment and which system's method of interpretation for triangle pose is the most "right." Personally, I have had heart-opening and mind-expanding experiences under the guidance of expert teachers, only to follow the session with a group analysis to reconstruct the sequence, rather than commune with the others regarding the sanctity of the experience or the depth of realization I have had. Rarely do I and my fellow practitioners just sit and simply enjoy one another in the silence of the state that follows practice. This phenomenon of reconstructing the sequence or debating the details occurs so commonly that I can only assume that it is symptomatic of being consumed by the temple's construction process, over and above the worship service that is going on inside the building. It is as though we have built a church with such intricate stained glass windows, beautiful mosaic tile designs and unique door handles that we actually forget to go inside and prostrate ourselves at the altar in prayer and thanksgiving.

Technique in asana is important, and like in any building project, form and function are inextricably linked. Taking time to construct each asana carefully is actually a kind of karma yoga, where our work to align is a devotional offering in and of itself. However, at a certain point, the building methods themselves should be taking us inward. Ideally, we would learn to follow the construction techniques to where they are designed to lead us—deeper into the sanctum sanctorum of the temple where we can expand and develop the inner architecture, our inner life.

Worship and Adoration

"At the heart of things, at the essence of things, all of this is the play of phenomena . . . At the heart of things there has never been any separation from Yogi Ramsuratkumar, only communion, *baraka*, benediction, grace. All the rest is the sparkling display of phenomena.

It is Shiva Nataraj—Shiva dancing out the play of phenomena. . . . [I]f we find ourselves in the play of phenomena, then the human thing to do is to be in that play according to God's design. At the heart of things everything is all the same. Everyone is the same regardless of color, caste, or religious belief. If one is a beggar, rich or poor, we are all the same. There is no present, past, future, time or space, only Father in Heaven. And yet, finding ourselves in this dance, it behooves us to play however the Divine Choreographer has written us into the dance.

So I have asked Yogi Ramsuratkumar to allow my sense of distinction to remain. In terms of an illusory prayer, I've asked Yogi Ramsuratkumar, in his grace, to allow me to be able to see myself as distinct from him so that I may bow at his feet in America. I have asked to remain in a mood of adoration or worship of him, because I find the state of adoration or worship to be the best state of all..."—Lee Lozowick, quoted in M. Young, *Yogi Ramsuratkumar, Under the Punnai Tree*, 518.

Question to Consider and Write About

What does it mean to you to develop the inner life of the temple of your body?

Beauty

> *Whatever being is endowed with beauty, goodness, glory and might, know that it has from a spark of my splendor.*
>
> —Bhagavad Gita *X.41*

We constantly receive distorted messages about beauty from the media today, and many of us find ourselves at the mercy of these distortions in the beliefs we hold to and the choices we make. In order to contemplate what real beauty is, it may be useful to familiarize ourselves with what beauty isn't.

I assert that real beauty often has little to do with anything Madison Avenue and its marketing machine tells us is beautiful. These images of false beauty abound and seduce us into their net of shallow concerns, sometimes at life-threatening costs. On the other hand, real beauty is that which takes us deeper into our hearts and reveals to us the genuine nature of reality. It initiates within us a mood of prayer and devotion. Developing a relationship with beauty involves, but is not limited to, learning to recognize, appreciate, praise, and create beauty in our many activities and endeavors, and for our purposes here, most specifically in asana, pranayama and mantra practice. Beauty is one of the primary ways that we begin to enliven the sanctuary of our inner life.

In the discussion of the tattvas in Chapter 11, we saw that the inner vehicle is made of three parts—the manas, which collects and perceives data and impressions through the sense organs and the organs of action, the ahamkara, which coordinates our sense of self or identity, and the buddhi, which is the higher aspect of intuition and spiritual awareness. You can imagine these three aspects working together in a somewhat linear way almost like a stepladder—with the manas on the bottom taking in data, the ahamkara sorting and using that data to create an identity, and the buddhi at the top, in some ways being an end result of our work on the rungs below it. Therefore, we can access the buddhi easier if we culture ourselves at the bottom rung according to these buddhi qualities.

A friend of mine had been sick with an autoimmune illness for almost a year when she attended an Anusara Yoga workshop with John Friend. He helped her overcome this illness through a skillful application of these principles—manas, ahamkara and buddhi. This woman told me that as John Friend was working with her, he began to talk to her and the whole group about what a great person she was. He described at length her beauty, her role in the community, and her great worth as a person. She said that so much positive attention was really making her uncomfortable. She felt tremendously awkward. Eventually, however, she told me that she simply surrendered to the affirmation, telling herself to just let it in. Almost immediately following that orientation of surrender, both she and John Friend looked at one another with the recognition that "It was gone." She was healed, and has had no reoccurrence of the symptoms that plagued her for almost a year.

When I heard this story I thought immediately of how interrelated the mind, the body, the emotions and our sense of self are. If, for instance, the ahamkara is weak, it actually becomes more subject to immune problems. The body is then a good host for disease. But, when the *ahamkara* is strong, certain viruses cannot thrive in the positive atmosphere that is informed by principles of beauty and truth. For instance, this student's healing came right after she surrendered to John Friend's affirmation of her essential beauty and worthiness. He clearly bolstered her ahamkara in the affirmation process and the illness was no longer at home in her system. Her system was different than it was when the virus had first taken hold of her.

While this is a striking example of the mind-body-emotions working together toward wellness or illness, I am not suggesting that every illness is a result of a weak sense of self or a lack of inner beauty or truth. That is much too bold a claim to make. But, if we look at self-hatred, self-doubt and its many manifestations of our low self-esteem as viruses or parasites, then this story serves as a most excellent illustration of a useful principle. How often are we actively attempting to make ourselves a poor host for the virus of self-hatred and self-destruction? How often are we consciously cultivating an inner atmosphere that will not host such negativity? Most of us spend more time making sure our computers are virus-free than worrying about whether our inner life has adequate virus protection!

Surrounding ourselves with beauty is one of the best virus-protection programs we can run. Sacred art such as iconographic statuary, uplifting music and mantra all feed the manas in positive ways. Good company, positive self-talk and our foundational and supportive practices all develop the ahamkara in a way that points us more readily toward the buddhi. In seeing this process through the metaphor of our temple building project, we can liken this process to interior decorating. We decorate the inner life according to principles of real beauty rather than the false ideals of our conditioning.

Questions to Consider and Write About

1. What is real beauty?
2. What viruses have a hold of you?
3. What virus protection might you run for yourself?

sixteen

Asana as Sacred Art

He has no canvas, brush, paints, stones, hammer or chisel, yet he chisels his own body with the asanas, develops the senses by ethics, stores energy through breath and with superb and supreme beauty tones the consciousness with the brilliance of the inner cosmic rays, or with the radiant light of his soul. He and his abode become one and henceforth the body becomes his heaven on earth.

—B.K.S. Iyengar

Sacred art is art that reminds us of the sacred, and is used for the purposes of worship and invocation. While any object of beauty has the ability to influence us and to invoke in us feelings of exaltation and reverence, sacred art's sole purpose is to radiate essential beauty in the form of sacred images so that we come into a state of resonance with the image and its meaning. In this state of resonance we are more able to recognize that same state of beauty in ourselves.

As we deepen our life of practice and establish ourselves more fully in the practices and principles of building a temple of the body, we use our asana practice as more than just a building project, more than just a set of techniques that we perform. Our practice becomes an act of creating sacred art.

In aligning ourselves with such a grand yet practical intention, we move into the inner life of the temple and prepare the inner chamber for worship. Like so much of this process, how asana becomes art is not so much in a set of fixed techniques as it is in one's attitude and intention for practice.

When I studied yoga in India several years ago, the teacher of the intensive began class one day talking about the poses as icons. He pointed to the different statues of Hindu deities throughout the yoga center. He said, I think for the benefit of what he assumed were mostly Judeo-Christian Westerners, "These statues are not idols; they are icons." I believe he was pointing to the idea that the imagery and the symbols used in the different statues actually held a certain power to transmit the sacred. These statues, as icons, were not simply mere representations or images as the word "idol" implies. The statues were actually *that which they represented*. This teacher went on to say that our poses should be approached as though they were icons.

Throughout much of India, the word *vigraha* refers to a statue of a deity in which the actual essence of the deity is believed to reside. A vigraha in the Hindu tradition differs from a mere statue or idol. It carries the essence of the saint or deity that it represents, and is regarded as the embodiment of the deity itself. For instance, placed in the center of Yogi Rmasuratkumar's temple is a huge statue of the saint himself, considered a vigraha. Today, this statue is worshipped *as* Yogi Ramsuratkumar and is seen as the very heart of his temple. Sacred iconographic art is extremely powerful. It also provides us with a clue about how we can use iconographic asana in a similar way in preparing our inner temple for worship.

An Impossible Task

On December 18, 1997 a larger than life statue of Yogi Ramsuratkumar cast in a dark bronze—a vigraha—was installed in the center of the . . . large temple. It had been in process for a few years, and was sculpted by Sri Kalasagar Rajagopal, the same sculptor who made the life-size statue of Ramana Maharshi at Ramanashram. The installation of the statue was a very important, auspicious event that caused a great deal of work for everyone.

Yogi Ramsuratkumar had been waiting for it to be done for some time. When the statue finally arrived, he declared that he wanted a permanent pedestal beneath the statue, and he told Mani that he wanted it installed without anyone touching the statue, which was now located in the middle of the temple. The workers listened to Mani in disbelief. How could such a thing be possible? The statue was almost three meters tall and weighed tons. The workers argued with Mani, who said, "you don't understand—Yogi Ramsuratkumar doesn't want the statue touched, so we will find a way to do it without touching the statue!" Somehow, it was done the way the master wanted it done." —M. Young, *Yogi Ramsuratkumar, Under the Punnai Tree*, 471-472.

Each pose has its own imagery, symbolism and its own ability to transmit an objective quality of the Divine. In other words, each pose can be approached as a work of sacred art. In any given asana practice, we assume the forms of geometric shapes, trees, birds, reptiles, animals, sages, saints and gods! Therefore, each pose can be approached as an artistic doorway into deeper understanding of yourself and the one consciousness that pervades every form.

In approaching asana as icons, as doorways from the finite to the Infinite, we are a long way from the discussion of the rights and wrongs of outer alignment. Instead, we have moved into the inner life of the practice, into the inner life of the temple, where each asana is both creative and decorative. Once we have some facility at outer form, we must take time to *be* in the pose. We must stop obsessively working on the poses and allow them to work on us; to reveal to us the wisdom inherent in their architecture and iconography. This wisdom often comes in the form of feeling or *bhavana*. Have you noticed that poses like *Virabhadrasana* 2 (warrior 2) have a different quality or feeling to them than *vrksasana* (tree pose) or *siddhasana* (adept's pose)? Their iconography is different. They are different images, designed to transmit different qualities to the practitioner. Just as a tree is quite different from Lord Shiva in his warrior's wrath, each pose is a different work of art. Through practice, attention and intention we can grow sensitive to the different teachings that each pose, as an icon, has to offer us.

Just as the asanas themselves have different moods and feeling qualities, the mood and feeling we bring to asana is paramount. For instance, we can approach the practice of asana from an artistic standpoint or a scientific standpoint. Consider how a scientist talks about the moon compared to how an artist or a poet describes the same heavenly body. As asana practitioners we can talk about the body, the asana, and our practice like a scientist talks about the moon—with measurements, technical terms and scientific facts. Or, we can be like a poet or an artist and approach our asana creatively through metaphor, inspiring imagery, and with the intention to see our efforts as artistic, devotional offerings.

Obviously, there is a time to be a scientist in asana. In my opinion there is also a time to be a bit of an athlete. But as we move into the inner life of the temple, as we expand our relationship with the universal spirit that lives within the temple we have built, we must cultivate the life of the mystical artist so that we are in the right frame of mind and heart for prayer and worship.

Approaching asana as sacred art is appropriate for all levels of practitioners, not only the physically adept. Obviously, as beginning artists, we might be less proficient in our skills and perhaps less masterful in the creative process, but asana as art is not attached to the outer performance of the posture. Approaching asana as an artist is linked first and foremost to attitude, mood and the intention to create beauty in a way that serves the heart's aim and creates within the temple of the body an atmosphere of refinement and sanctity.

Questions to Consider and Write About

1. What does it mean to you to practice asana as art?
2. Do you typically approach asana as a scientist, an athlete or a mystic?

seventeen

Pranayama as an Invocational Dance

Pranayama is often defined as "control of the breath" or "control of the life force" (prana). The word has two parts: *prana*, meaning "life force" and *yama*, meaning "control" or "restraint." However, if we divide the word just a little differently its nuances change considerably. After all, *pran* means "life force" and *ayama* means "expansion." Pranayama, for the purposes of building a temple of the body, can best be understood as "expansion of the life force" rather than the *control* of it.

The entire list of benefits of pranayama practice are too numerous to include here. But, to name a few:

- Physiologically, pranayama is an excellent way to keep our inner sanctuary clean, pure and enlivened. It is as though we can, through practice, bring the breath and our awareness into the interior chambers of the temple of the body to cleanse and sweep out any accumulated toxins.
- Emotionally and mentally, pranayama helps us stabilize our moods and our reactions by balancing our nervous system more optimally and training us to

> live with greater awareness and attention. By practicing pranayama we become more exquisitely aware of our own inner architecture.

The technology of pranayama is immense and can be quite demanding. Yet even with the best technique, pranayama without devotion becomes dry and devoid of its rich transformational potential.

Pranayama is best practiced with a mood of devotional introspection in which the practitioner seeks expansion, over and above control or domination. When the practice of pranayama is pursued with regularity and with devotion, pranayama is more like a creative, invocational dance that occurs in the inner chambers of our own temple than a mere set of breathing exercises.

In the *Anusara Yoga Teacher Training Manual*, John Friend has described the optimal context for pranayama in this way:

> Ultimately we are not in control of the breath. The breath is the movement of the Goddess. She exhales into us when we are born and inhales Herself completely out of us when we die. We are actually being breathed by a greater power. We cannot govern the vast energy behind the breath by natural means. For example, if you try to kill yourself by holding you breath, you will eventually pass out and your breathing will start automatically.
>
> She is the lead dancer of life, seeking a dance partner in us. If we follow in harmony with the natural movements of the breath, we can participate in the creation of a magical and wondrous dance with Her. Breathing should be considered a sacred and divine

honor. It is as if the greatest dancer of all time comes to ask you to dance with Her—an incredible honor! With this understanding, you breathe with great humility, care and joy. You let the master dancer lead the way, and you follow as best you can so that the dance appears as one singular expression of harmony and joy. Thus, instead of trying to be ultimately in charge of the breath, we should simply dance with Her.

This cooperative, humble attitude is one of the major tenets of Anusara Yoga. There is no attempt to control, dominate or subjugate Nature. There are four main points to remember while we dance and breathe with The Goddess:

—Open to Grace.

—Ultimately, we are not in control.

—The movement of *prana* inside us is the Grace of the Goddess. She wants to enter us, so we simply have to open ourselves up to receive Her. She waits for us until we can cultivate enough trust and courage to open up freely to Her greater power.

—Instead of trying to pull Her into your lungs on inhalation, simply open the ribs and lungs and welcome Her.[(1)]

When engaged from this context of creative participation, pranayama becomes one of the most powerful practices we have to expand our relationship with the universal aspect of ourselves and the inner life of the temple of the body. Inspiration and expiration, words that refer to inhaling and exhaling, both share the same root, *-spire*, which means "spirit" or "soul." This etymological correlation gives us a clue to what the yogis have known all along—that the breath most certainly links us to the life of the spirit. By expanding our relationship with the breath through pranayama, we can expand our relationship with the spirit or soul that lives at the heart of the temple of the body. We can dance in prayer and offering to the spirit that inhabits our great temple.

On a practical note, pranayama, like other practices, is most effective when practiced regularly. Experiment with what time of day you are most likely to practice pranayama with the most consistency, and make a commitment to a set period of time for pranayama practice. Remember that *most* people find themselves distractible, and often bored and frustrated, in the early stages of pranayama practice. If, however, in the midst of these obstacles, we can reassert our intention, establish ourselves in the optimal context and persevere, the rewards are worth the struggle.

Questions to Consider and Write About

1. What does your pranayama practice consist of now?
2. How might the idea of "expanding the life force" rather than controlling it affect your pranayama practice positively?

eighteen

Mantra as Devotional Music: Changing Your Background Noise

Mantras start a powerful vibration which corresponds to both a specific spiritual energy frequency and a state of consciousness in seed form. Over time, the mantra process begins to override all of the other smaller vibrations, which eventually become absorbed by the mantra. After a length of time which varies from individual to individual, the great wave of the mantra stills all other vibrations. Ultimately, the mantra produces a state where the organism vibrates at the rate completely in tune with the energy and spiritual state represented by and contained within the mantra.

—Thomas Ashley-Farrard

Wouldn't it be shocking if you walked into a temple to pray and instead of uplifting, heart-oriented music playing on the organ there was loud, heavy-metal music blasting through the sound system with messages of death, destruction and violence? Obviously, that would seem out of sync with your intention for going to the temple in the first place. But for many of us, the background noise of our inner lives is similar to what I just described. Oftentimes, the music playing in our temple is a litany of complaints, judgments, criticisms, worries and projections. Mantra, the repetition of sacred sounds, is a great way to create a type of background noise for our inner sanctuary that is more optimal than our usual self-talk.

The science of mantra is, obviously, much more refined than creating new background noise. In fact, some of the earliest yoga scriptures, The Vedas, "maintain that everything comes into being through the power of speech. Ideas remain un-actualized until they are created through the power of speech."(1) The power of our spoken words, whether those words are spoken out loud or expressed within the privacy of our own thoughts, determines much of how we see the world and our place in it. If we want to expand the inner life of our temple so that the atmosphere within us is conducive to worship, we will benefit from the practice of mantra.

In the spiritual school of which I am a part, we use Yogi Ramsuratkumar's name as our primary mantra. He gave this practice to his devotees saying that: "If someone repeats this beggar's name he will be helping the work of this beggar, he will be helping the world, and he will be helping himself. You repeat the name of this mad fellow then I will be with you." And again: "Yogi Ramsuratkumar is not the name of this beggar . . . Yogi Ramsuratkumar is the name of my Father."(2)

If the word or concept of mantra seems foreign or esoteric to you, it might help to think about mantras as prayers or as affirmations. It is not necessary to use a Sanskrit mantra (although they can be quite helpful) if that makes you feel uncomfortable. But learning to align your inner monologue with your heart's intention is a real way to change the music you are playing inside yourself.

The Universe of God's Name

"Another unique characteristic of Bhagavan is to make devotees of other great Mahatmas to sing the praise of their respective gurus. When the devotees of Sri Ramana come to Him, He will make them sing songs on Bhagavan Ramana, discuss about Ramana and make them read several times articles on or passages from Ramana. When the devotees of Sri Ramakrishna come, He will make them speak of the Trinity—Sri Ramakrishna, Holy Mother Sri Sarada and Swami Vivekanand—and hear with devotion their narrations. When a devotee of Pagal Harnath comes, Bhagavan will speak about Harnath. Once a devotee of J. Krishnamoorthy asked Bhagavan to give him a photo of Bhagavan. Bhagavan simply told the devotee to follow the path of J.K. steadfastly. I have enjoyed seeing Him dance in ecstasy, singing 'Om Sri Ram jai Ram jai Jai Ram,' along with devotees of Anandashram. To the devotees of Sri Satya Sai Baba, He would ask for Sai Bhajans and make them read the Guru-poornima lecture of Sri Satya Sai Baba and hail it as the 'Voice of God.'" —Ma Devaki, quoted in Regina Sara Ryan, *Only God, A Biography of Yogi Ramsuratkumar*, 521.

As with pranayama, it can be helpful to practice mantra in a formal, ritualized way with regularity. I personally begin my morning with pranayama, followed by my mantra practice and then with a period of meditation. During the mantra practice I begin by repeating the mantra out loud, then silently to myself, and then I take my attention deeper inward to penetrate the power of the energy within the words themselves. While other techniques for mantra can be employed, the main point here is that by taking the time to formally practice mantra, you will establish a resonance to the practice and to the mantras that you are using. This energetic resonance will strengthen the effects of the mantra so that the background noise of the sanctuary will be made conscious, uplifting and aligned with your highest purpose.

Questions to Consider and Write About

1. What is your current background noise?
2. What music would you like to be playing in the temple of your body?

PART V

WORSHIP: LIFE AT THE SHRINE OF THE HEART

Worship, together with expressions of gratitude, love, communion and devotion . . . these and other interior attitudes and activities are awakened in us through our yoga practice. In this part we will approach with reverence to the "holy of holies," the shrine that lies deep within the body, at the very heart of the temple.

nineteen

Darshan of the Heart

The soul, smaller than the small, greater than the great,
is hidden in the hearts of all living creatures.
—Katha Upanishad

When two opposing forces are balanced, the place of balance is called "the middle." The teachings of Kashmir Shaivism suggest that when opposites are in their optimal relationship of creative tension, an opening of the heart occurs. As yoga practitioners we are continually instructed to balance effort with ease, freedom with discipline, zeal with detachment, and so on. These pairs of opposites are at the heart of building a temple of the body. In order for balance to characterize our inner life as it relates to our temple-building project, our particular notion of balance must be mature, not confused with some new-age ideas or notions. We are not looking for a balanced state where some bland middle ground of calm suddenly descends upon us. We are, more accurately, entering into a dynamic relationship where two ends of a spectrum are brought together with an appropriate amount of creative tension so that transformation, or perhaps more accurately *revelation*, occurs. This dynamic tension is sometimes described as a "pulsation," "vibration" or even a "throb." The philosophers of Kashmir Shaivism called it *spanda*. The pulsing, throbbing quality that we see throughout the manifested world—inhalation and exhalation, night and day, eyes opening and eyes closing—are simply microcosmic reflections of the nature of the Divine. Throbbing in its fullness, the Divine exists as creative tension itself. When we practice balance skillfully, when we participate consciously in bringing opposing forces together—in asana, in marriage, in our vocation—we are establishing ourselves in a relationship with spanda, with the Divine pulse itself.

The word *mudya* in Sanskrit means "the middle." *Mudya* also means "heart," "center," and therefore could mean "that which is at the heart of the matter." At the heart of the matter, it seems, is the heart itself. When we are stable in a place of expansion, we glimpse the inner chamber of the heart where two apparent opposites exist simultaneously without conflict, and where we exist in the "tension between the opposites" at the shrine of our hearts, at the source of our own creative potential.

Shrine of the Heart

At the heart of any temple is an altar or shrine that serves as a focal point for ceremonial prayer and ritual worship. Each of us who wishes to create a temple of the body will want to erect such a shrine within ourselves to serve as a place of refuge and renewal. Some yogic texts have called this place the "cave of the heart" and have described a small being the size of a thumb who is seated there doing ritual prayer. When I first heard this teaching I was immediately struck by the idea that, just as the alignment of asana is not an imposition *on* the body but an alignment *with* an optimal blueprint, a life of prayer and devotion is not an imposition either. A devotional life is simply bringing ourselves into alignment with this aspect of self who is already seated at the shrine of our hearts worshipping and praying.

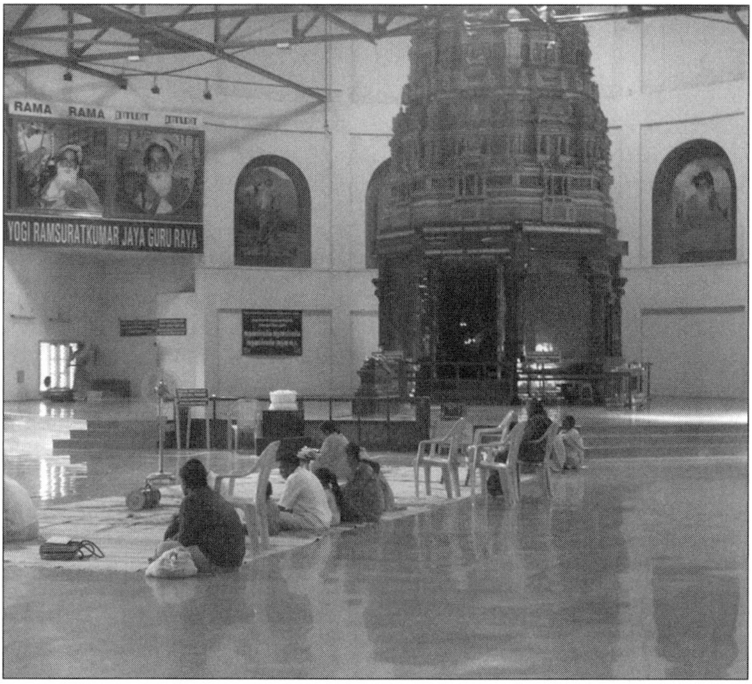

Devotees chant within the temple, close to the samadhi shrine of Yogi Ramsuratkumar, 2010.

For the purposes of metaphoric consistency I will proceed in this section calling this inner chamber "the shrine" rather than the cave of the heart. Ultimately, the exact imagery we use is not so important. What is important is that each of us develops an active relationship with a place of worship within; a place that is not dependent on time, location or circumstance. In this inner chamber healing occurs, insight arises and the aim of yoga is realized. To this altar we come to worship, pray and seek what Lee Lozowick has often called, the "darshan of the heart."

Darshan is a Sanskrit word derived from the root *darś-*, which means "to see." Darshan means "sight," "vision," "apparition," or "glimpse" in the sense of an instance of seeing or beholding.

Darshan most commonly refers to "visions of the divine"—as in a god, holy person or artifact. One could "receive the darshana" of the deity in the temple, or from a great saintly person, such as a great guru.

Throughout the yoga traditions we find references to the seat of the self being in the heart of each of us. The darshan of the heart, then, means to have an audience with our truest self—that which is at the center of who we are. Darshan of the heart means to see and to be seen from the heart's truth. It is in glimpsing this truth that we are forever changed. We are transformed. We are no longer the same person who first broke ground and struggled to lay a solid foundation. Certainly we can repeat old patterns, and most likely we will. Change does not mean that we are suddenly free of all of our bad habits and idiosyncratic behaviors. We are most certainly not suddenly free from the need to keep practicing according to dharmic principles. Being changed by the darshan of the heart means that we have expanded so that, even if we contract again, our capacity has been increased forever. We are not the same.

Recently I was struggling with some of my own doubts relative to my sadhana and spiritual path. I sought the council of my mentor who listened carefully and thoughtfully. When I asked her for feedback she said simply, "Well, at some point, you just realize that the guru has moved into your heart. And try as you might to get him to, he is not going to leave." That teaching illustrates my point exactly. At a certain point we are changed, and the old—be it ideas, behaviors, dreams and/or relationships—while we may revisit them occasionally, just do not fit the same way they used to.

This is the boon of the darshan of the heart. But this boon asks of us as much as it gives to us. We must take this gift of seeing into our lives so that we begin to see the world from the heart's perspective. Our task at this stage of the temple-building project is to stabilize our heart's expansion. We can learn to be stable and established in this expanded view of the heart. We can grow stable in this new way of seeing so that we are functional and possess equanimity in the expanded view that the darshan of the heart provides. And, as much as the darshan of heart is essentially an inside job, the darshan of the heart occurs anytime we are willing to see and to be seen through the eyes of love. Any time we let others love us, any time we choose a loving response, we are worshipping at the shrine of the heart.

As we grow fuller and more skillful in our new perspective, we begin to see, sometimes quickly and sometimes slowly, that the darshan of the heart has been guiding us all along. We have been drawn inward, in numerous ways and through various means, to the recesses of our heart by that self inside who is praying and constantly offering puja.

Questions to Consider and Write About

1. What is the darshan of the heart?
2. When have you experienced seeing yourself through the eyes of the heart?
3. In what ways is this perspective difficult for you?

twenty

Communion

Meditate on your own Self.
Worship your Self.
Respect your Self.
God dwells within you as you.
—Swami Muktananda

Central to the Christian tradition is the ceremony of the Holy Eucharist or Holy Communion, a ritual that most of us have at least heard about, if not participated in, at some point in our lives. This ritual is an affirmation of the covenant between Jesus and his disciples, and they with him. Many of the Indian guru traditions, which inform various yoga schools and esoteric sects, engage in similar rituals of communion with the exchange of *prasad*.

Prasad, meaning "divine gift," is exchanged between the master and the devotee and symbolizes the reciprocal relationship or covenant in which they are engaged. While these explanations are reasonably simple and straightforward, these ceremonies are the exterior enactment of a deep inner connectedness. Implicit in these ceremonies is the mood of communion—of coming into union with the Divine. Disciples of Christ—both modern and historical—experience the Divine

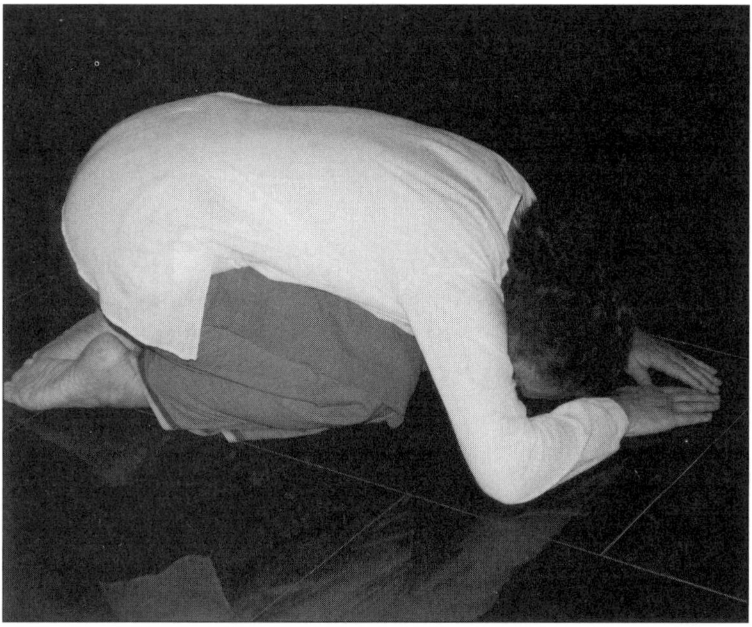

Lee Lozowick bows to his guru, Yogi Ramsuratkumar

through the form and teachings of Jesus Christ, who serves as a doorway to the kingdom of heaven that is within. To disciples or devotees of a guru, communion is experienced through the door of the guru. Other traditions certainly have their equivalent rituals and ceremonies, and many people develop their own personal rituals to experience communion.

Essentially, communion with any outer image is there to assist us in experiencing communion with the inner Beloved—that aspect of the Divine that is within us *as us*. In the Bhagavad Gita, there are references to the idea that people can and will successfully relate to the Divine in different ways, some personal, others impersonal.(1) The Beloved is a personal way to relate to the Absolute. I have found that while people's faiths and religions vary, and therefore their concepts of the Absolute may vary slightly, people of most faiths relate to the idea of the "Beloved." In my experience, a mood of softening arises when people consider the Beloved. As personal as the concept is, it also seems to be quite universal.

As an author and a teacher I am uninterested in determining for anyone how they personally engage the Beloved. I am, however, a passionate believer in the importance of establishing ourselves in such a relationship. The idea of the Beloved comes to its fullness in the devotional yoga traditions called *bhakti yoga*, whose emphasis was not so much on *overcoming* separation, like many yoga schools, but on *staying* "separated" for the purposes of being able to love and worship. Think about it—from the state of union, there is no "other" to love. The only way to love and to worship another is when we are separate from them. Certainly, through the practices of devotion a union or joining occurs, but the great gift of the perception of separation is that it enables us to worship, to praise, to pray and to experience ourselves in relationship to the Beloved.

One of the ways that we stabilize the expansion of the heart is to recognize the source of the darshan of the heart and to enter into communion with the Beloved of our heart. When we are connected so deeply to our source, we are no longer at the mercy of life's ups and downs, the winds of change, and the fickle tides of public opinion. Rather, we are seated, in prayer and worship at the shrine of the heart, in communion with the Beloved. It does not get more stable than that.

> . . . There is only You, Beloved, only You,
>   no second, no separation, no confusion,
> no misunderstanding, no question, ever.
>   Once lee met You, all else faded into
> complete emptiness beside the substance
>   of Your Heart and Your Oneness, Your Blessing.
>
> —lee lozowick
> 14 January 2000[(2)]

PART VI

OUTREACH MINISTRY: CELEBRATION THROUGH SERVICE

In this final chapter we return our attention to where we started in our temple-buiding project—to our intention to serve and to offer our efforts to what lies beyond our personal aims and desires. Truly, the power of yoga practice is not in what it does for us personally but in what it allows us to do for others.

twenty-one

Service and Outreach

My yoga isn't about liberation . . . it's about becoming a perfect vehicle for the service of God.

—Yogi Ramsuratkumar

I consciously avoided ending this book with a section about adding a ceiling or a steeple to the temple. My teacher Lee Lozowick has always said that there is "no top end" in terms of sadhana and practice, and so our temple-building project must remain a bit open ended as well. While we will always have building maintenance and even some restoration projects to do as time goes by, we must dedicate ourselves *now* to service and outreach.

In the section on intention, Chapter 1, we noted that when Yogi Ramsuratkumar built his temple he did not begin the project thinking it would be fun, or a way for him to entertain himself or stay busy. He began with only one reason in mind—that his temple would serve to transmit his blessings for generations to come. The same intention applies to our building a temple of the body. Hopefully, it will be a monument to and for the great architect who will work through us to uplift, heal and minister to those in need.

Certainly, people come to yoga initially as a way to take care of themselves, and some folks practice yoga because going to classes fills a social need. The reasons why people practice are broad and varied, and generally all of these reasons are great! Rarely do I hear a reason that seems even a bit questionable to me. (Have you ever heard someone say, "I practice yoga to gain power and control over others"?!) Physical health, psychological well-being and every personal benefit we could name as an outcome of yoga practice are great and wonderful things. But, if those personal benefits stop with us, if the temple we have built becomes merely a monument to ourselves, then we have missed the point of yoga. Ultimately, it's all about service.

As much as it strengthens and stretches our bodies, yoga should be strengthening and stretching our capacity to love ourselves and one another. Yoga, additionally, is about strengthening and stretching our ability to serve this love. If we are not more able, as result of yoga practice, to sacrifice our personal comfort occasionally in the name of the love we feel, then our personal "Department of Outreach Ministry" needs a new team leader!

The Nature of Service

"[Yogi Ramsuratkumar] had said once that even fishing in the sea was sadhana if it were offered to God. He had warned that we should not vie for big changes or targets to be reached. Do not try to become a sage, seer, or saint. Try to become a simple soul for others as divine service. Simple is always beautiful; humbleness is a great quality. 'There is no more achievement once you come into the company of this beggar,' he said many times.

"Bhagwan told me that His Father had chosen me and blessed me to do his Father's work. It was He who had shown me to the path of karma yoga. It was my work that I offered to Him, to God. And in conducting my work for Bhagwan, I had to decide over and chose over and over again not to worry or waste precious, blessed time with my work. My attention was to be on Bhagwan and what He was commanding of me—that was the nature of my own sadhana."—Mani, *A Man and His Master*, 154-155.

True Service

Not to be confused with martyrdom, co-dependency, obligation, or a lack of self-regard in which we put others first because we feel unworthy, true service is about allowing ourselves to be used as an agent of the Highest in the world. St. Teresa of Avila, in the fourteenth century, spoke of this idea when she said that "God has no hands but our hands" to do his work today. We erected our temple, we cultivated our body of practice, not for our own ends but so that we could be God's hands in the world. We did the work so that we could have the privilege of sharing in the tasks that need to be done. Service was the point all along.

The path of true service can be tricky because so often our notion of service is based on our assumptions, projections and ideas of what would help, rather than on what is truly wanted and needed. Many times, as we are learning the art of service, we are bound to try to help in ways that actually hinder. It takes sensitivity, clarity and practice to serve optimally, just as it takes a long time to learn certain yoga poses. As tricky a path as it is to walk, service is, in my opinion, what yoga is actually about.

In its truest form, service is not so much about continually putting our needs aside as about truly having fewer needs to begin with. Often, what we consider our needs are actually ways to buffer ourselves from a sense of emptiness, isolation and discomfort. As we grow in sadhana, our ability to navigate this uncomfortable psychological territory improves, and many of our needs are not what we thought they were. This recognition, however, cannot be forced. It is an outcome of practice. Optimal service arises from a place of spiritual fullness where we are no longer as dependent on creature comforts, external affirmation and outside gratification because we have fed the true sources of those needs and hungers through practice over a long period of time.

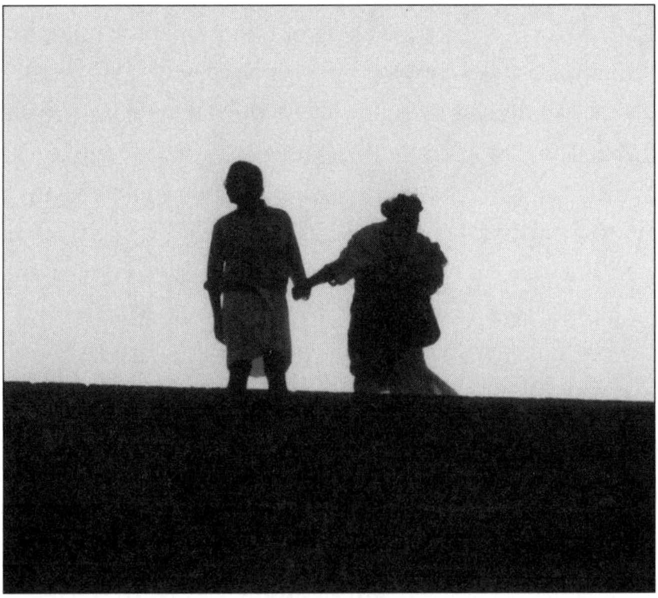

Yogi Ramsuratkumar holds Mani's hand, 1994.

Small Gestures, Here and Now

Serving others is sometimes grand in scale. But for most of us, service lives in small gestures of kindness, compassion and generosity. Service is the extension of attitude into the world; and attitude that is optimally aligned and skillfully expressed in the world is one of the most attractive forces in the universe, literally magnetic in nature. This attitude will attract to us people, circumstances and situations so that our desire to serve and to share our heart's fullness will be put to use.

Serving others happens right where we are, through us *as we are*. We do not need to wait until we are perfect, without fault and fully evolved to extend our hearts and hands lovingly in service. In fact, by sharing our imperfections and struggles honestly with one another, we may serve by demonstrating compassion and understanding that puts an end to feelings of isolation and self-judgment.

How we serve is not as important as *that* we serve. If we begin each day by establishing our resolve to be "God's hands in the world," I believe we will begin to see numerous service opportunities arise in each moment.

God *As* You

I often imagine that if I were God and I was looking out onto my creation, I would see the suffering, the competition, the jealousy, the violence, the degradation and the true need for compassionate responses. Observing this great need, I wouldn't be so picky about whom I put to work. In fact, I would give jobs to just about anybody who raised their hand sincerely wanting to help out. Those people who were able to help in big ways, I would push to their limits. Those more restricted in capacity, I would push to their limits as well. People who love nature I would assign to helping the earth. People who loved animals I would assign to work with animals. People who felt for the children, I would surround with children. And so on. I would assign people, based on their interest, capacity, talents and drives to help anywhere they could or would help.

Let's face it, there is tremendous need in the world; great suffering everywhere we look. No act of service, then, is too small. And the best part is that in helping, in serving, we are served. We are participating in the work of the Divine. There is no higher privilege.

In her message for 2000, Gurumayi Chidvilasananda spoke about "uninterrupted loving service" as a way to dissolve that which separates us from the constant experience of Divine love. As we cultivate an attitude of service, we learn how to make all of our life's work service to God; all aspects of our life become yoga. Ultimately, we come to understand that serving humanity and serving God are one and the same.[(1)]

Having constructed a temple of the body through which to serve, we return to the first principle of putting the Highest first. We come full circle. Service leads us back to our original intention for the temple building project—to become a vehicle for and an expression of the Divine in the world. This body, with all of its frailties and challenges, with its unique strengths and capacities, is our body of practice, our consecrated temple and our means to engage the yoga of service.

May the temple that we call our body, and the body of practice that we call our life, be a place of refuge, sanctuary and inspiration for ourselves and all who are in need.

Appendix—The Tattvas

The 36 Tattvas of Tantric Cosmology Chart

The Absolute Tattvas

The Universal - Ultimate Reality

Macrocosmic Consciousness

Paramshiva

1. **Shiva** — Supreme Consciousness

2. **Shakti** — Power of Consciousness

3. **Sadashiva** — Iccha — willpower

4. **Isvara** — Jnana — knowledge

5. **Suddhavidya** — Kriya — action

Sat-Cit-Ānanda

Being-Consciousness-Bliss

Psychical Tattvas

Microcosmic Consciousness

6. **Māyā** - differentiating power of the universe

5 Kanchukas - Cloaks

7. **Kalā** - limits omnipotence (Kriya), creates limited agency or the capacity to act
8. **Vidya** - limits omniscience (Jnana) creates limited knowledge
9. **Raga** - limits fullness of heart; (Iccha) creates desire and longing to be full again
10. **Niyati** - limits omnipresence freedom of creative power and expression (Shakti) creates fabric of Space, and the energetic tapestry of casuality
11. **Kāla** - limits eternal awareness (Shiva) creates time, and the sense of sequential awareness

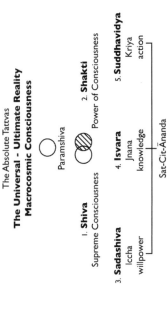

Physical Tattvas

The Relative World

12. **Purusha**
Male Principle

13. **Prakriti**
Female Principle

14. **Buddhi** - intelligence
15. **Ahamkāra** - ego sense
16. **Manas** - mental functions

Jnanendriyas
Five sense organs

17. **Ears** - auditory, hearing
18. **Skin** - tactile, feeling, touch
19. **Eyes** - visual, seeing
20. **Tongue** - gustatory, tasting
21. **Nose** - olfactory, smelling

Karmendriyas
Five action organs

22. **Mouth** - speaking
23. **Hands** - touching
24. **Feet** - ambulating
25. **Genitals** - procreating
26. **Bowels** - eliminating

Tanmatras
Five subtle elements

27. **Shabda** - Energy of vibration (sound-as-such)
28. **Sparsha** - Energy of Impact (touch-as-such)
29. **Rūpa** - Energy of light and form (form-as-such)
30. **Rasa** - Energy of viscous attraction (taste-as-such)
31. **Gandha** - Energy of cohesive attraction (smell-as-such)

Mahabhutas
Five gross elements

32. **Space** (Ākāsha)
33. **Air** (Vāyu)
34. **Fire** (Agni)
35. **Water** (Ap)
36. **Earth** (Prithivi)

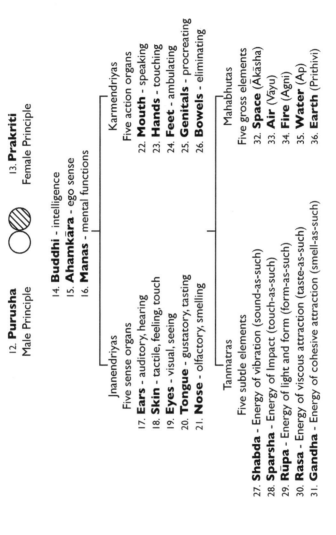

Tantric Tattva Correspondences Chart

Tattva	Subject/Object	Supreme Attribute	Kanchuchas
Shiva - Supreme Consciousness	I	Eternity	Kāla - Time
Shakti - Creative Power of the Supreme	AM	Omnipresence/ Freedom	Niyati - Space
Iccha - Divine Will	I AM This	Purna - Fullness	Raga - Desire
Jnana - Divine Knowledge	This I AM	Omniscience	Vidya - Limited Knowledge
Kriya - Divine Action	This and I	Omnipotence	Kāla - Limited Agency

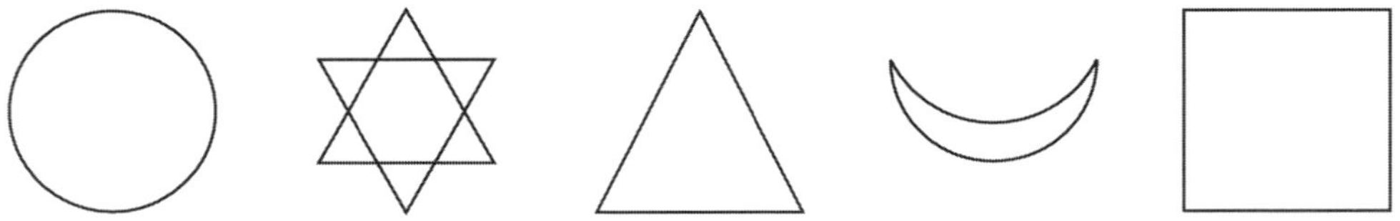

Sky Air Fire Water Earth

Tattva	5 Elements	3 Malas	3 Doshas
Shiva - Supreme Consciousness	Sky		
Shakti - Creative Power of the Supreme	Earth		
Iccha - Divine Will	Water	Anava	Kapha
Jnana - Divine Knowledge	Fire	Mayiya	Pitta
Kriya - Divine Action	Air	Karma	Vata

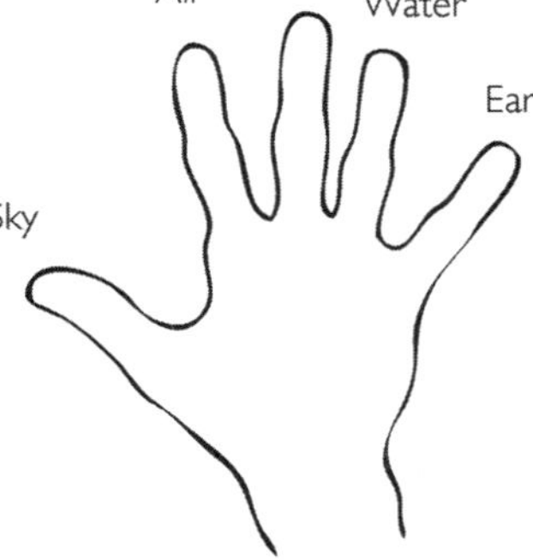

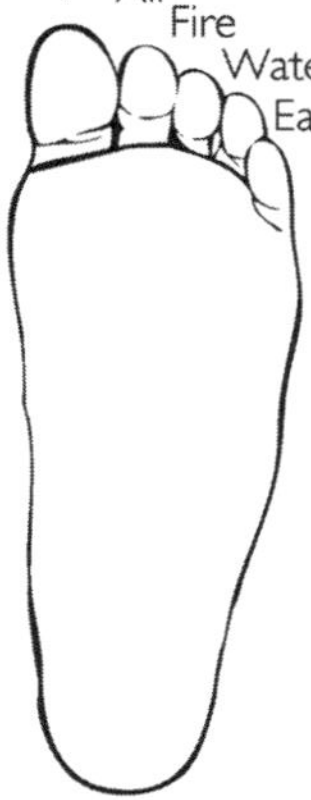

Jnanendriyas	Karmendriyas	Tanmatras	Mahabhutas
Ears	Mouth / speaking	Shabda - sound	Space
Skin	Hands / touching	Sparsha - touch	Air
Eyes	Feet / ambulating	Rụpa - color	Fire
Tongue	Genitals / procreating	Rasa - flavor	Water
Nose	Bowels / eliminating	Gandha - smell	Earth

Endnotes

Introduction

1. Iyengar, B.K.S., *Light on the Yoga Sutras of Patanjali.* (London: Thorsons, 1996), 53.
2. Personal correspondence.

2. The Highest First

1. Friend, John, *Anusara Yoga Teacher Training Manual.* (The Woodlands, Texas: Anusara Press, 1998), 20.
2. Brooks, Douglas lecture notes, quoted in: Christina Sell, *Yoga From the Inside Out: Making Peace with Your Body Through Yoga.* (Prescott, Arizona: Hohm Press, 2003), 78.
3. Friend, *Anusara Yoga Teacher Training Manual*, 18.
4. Iyengar, B.K.S., as quoted in public classes.
5. Quoted in: John Friend, *Immersion Curriculum Booklet* (The Woodlands, Texas: Anusara Press, 2006), 6.

4. Intrinsic Goodness

1. Rumbaugh, Desiree, personal correspondence.
2. Stephen, a student, personal correspondence.
3. Pomeda, Carlos, personal correspondence.

5. The Body

1. Feuerstein, Georg, *Tantra: The Path of Ecstasy.* (Boston, Mass.: Shambhala, 1998), 2.

2. Lecture notes, Carlos Pomeda on file.
3. Lecture notes, Dr. Stephen Phillips, personal correspondence.

6. Asking the Right Questions

1. John, Friend, *Immersion Curriculum Booklet*. (The Woodlands, Texas: Anusara Press, 2006), 9.

7. Attention

1. Mani with S. Lhaksam, *A Man and His Master*. (Prescott, Arizona: Hohm Press, 2004), 177.

9. Yamas and Niyamas

1. Pomeda, Carlos, lecture notes
2. Friend, John, *Anusara Yoga Teacher Training Manual*. (The Woodlands, Texas: Anusara Press, 1998), 87.
3. Ibid., 87-88.

10. The Conditions

1. Hohm Community, *Hohm Sahaj Mandir Study Manual*. (Prescott, Arizona: Hohm Press, 1996), 389-390.
2. Lozowick, Lee, quoted in: *Hohm Sahaj Mandir Study Manual*. (Prescott, Arizona: Hohm Press, 1996), 396.
3. Ibid., 405.
4. Ibid. 424-425.
5. Ibid. 427.

11. The Dharma

1. Iyengar, B.K.S., *Light on the Yoga Sutras of Patanjali*. (San Francisco, Calif.: Harper Collins, 1993), 3.

2. Iyengar, B.K.S., *Light on Life*. (Rodale Press, 2006), 240.
3. Singh, Jaideva. *Shiva Sutras The Yoga of Supreme Identity*. (Delhi: Motilal Banarsidass, 1979), v-xv.

12. Spiritual Authority and the Guru

1. Pomeda, Carlos, personal correspondence.
2. Ibid.
3. Ibid.
4. Feuerstein, Georg, *The Yoga Tradition*. (Hohm Press: Prescott, Arizona, 1998), 14.
5. Lozowick, Lee, quoted in: *Trimurti Journal*: *Who's Rowing Your Boat?* Volume XII February 2008. (Trimurti Ashram: Bozeman, Montana.)
6. Lozowick, Lee, quoted in: *Tawagoto*, *The Sacred Foolish Song of the Hohm Community*, Fall 1995, Vol.8, No.4, 52.
7. Friend, John, quoted in: Sell, Christina, *Yoga From The Inside Out: Making Peace with your Body Through Yoga*. (Prescott, Arizona: Hohm Press, 2003), 118-120.

13. The Kula

1. Mani, *A Man and His Master*. (Hohm Press: Prescott, Arizona, 2003), 178.
2. Lozowick, Lee, lecture notes.
3. Personal notes, on file.
4. Personal notes, on file.

14. Enthusiastic Discipline

1. Avalon, Arthur, *Kularnava Tantra*. (Delhi: Motilal Banarsidass, 2000), 36.

17. Pranayama as an Invocational Dance

1. Friend, John, *Anusara Yoga Teacher Training Manual.* (The Woodlands, Texas: Anusara Press, 1998), 52.

18. Mantra as Devotional Music

1. www.sanskritmantra.com Retrieved 03/12/08
2. Yogi Ramsuratkumar, quoted in Regina Sara Ryan, *Only God: A Biography of Yogi Ramsuratkumar*, (Prescott, Arizona: Hohm Press, 2004), 139.

20. Communion

1. Pomeda, Carlos, lecture notes.
2. Lozowick, Lee, *Gasping for Air in a Vacuum: Poems and Prayers to Yogi Ramsuratkumar*, (Prescott, Arizona: Hohm Press, 2004), excerpt from 444-445.

21. Service and Outreach

1. www.siddhayoga.com

Additional References

Mani, with S. Lhaksham, *A Man and His Master: My Years with Yogi Ramsuratkumar*, Prescott, Arizona: Hohm Press, 2003.

Ryan, Regina Sara, *Only God, A Biography of Yogi Ramsuratkumar*, Prescott, Arizona, 2004.

Young, Mary. *Yogi Ramsuratkumar: Under the Punnai Tree.* Prescott, Arizona: Hohm Press, 2003.

Index

A

B

C

G

H

I

J

K

L

M

S

V

W

Y

Z